TRAUMA-SENSITIVE YOGA

of related interest

Yoga Therapy for Parkinson's Disease and Multiple Sclerosis
Jean Danford
ISBN 978 1 84819 299 7
eISBN 978 0 85701 249 4

Yoga for a Happy Back
A Teacher's Guide to Spinal Health through Yoga Therapy
Rachel Krentzman, PT, E-RYT
Foreword by Aadil Palkhivala
ISBN 978 1 84819 271 3
eISBN 978 0 85701 253 1

Trauma is Really Strange
Steve Haines
Art by Sophie Standing
ISBN 978 1 84819 293 5
eISBN 978 0 85701 240 1

TRAUMA-SENSITIVE
YOGA

DAGMAR HÄRLE

FOREWORD BY DAVID EMERSON
TRANSLATED BY CHRISTINE M. GRIMM

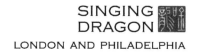

SINGING
DRAGON
LONDON AND PHILADELPHIA

First published in 2015 as 'Körperorientierte Traumatherapie: Sanfte Heilung
mit traumasensitivem Yoga' by Junfermann Verlag, Paderborn
This English language edition first published in 2017
by Singing Dragon
an imprint of Jessica Kingsley Publishers
73 Collier Street
London N1 9BE, UK
and
400 Market Street, Suite 400
Philadelphia, PA 19106, USA

www.singingdragon.com

Library of Congress Cataloging in Publication Data
Names: Härle, Dagmar, author.
Title: Trauma-sensitive yoga / Dagmar Härle ; foreword by David Emerson ;
    translated by Christine M. Grimm.
Other titles: Körperorientierte Traumatherapie. English
Description: English language edition. | London ; Philadelphia : Jessica
    Kingsley Publishers, 2017. | Includes bibliographical references and index.
Identifiers: LCCN 2016057252 | ISBN 9781848193468 (alk. paper)
Subjects: LCSH: Psychic trauma--Physical therapy. | Yoga--Therapeutic use.
Classification: LCC RC552.T7 H3713 2017 | DDC 616.85/21062--dc23
LC record available at https://lccn.loc.gov/2016057252

British Library Cataloguing in Publication Data
A CIP catalogue record for this book is available from the British Library

ISBN 978 1 84819 346 8
eISBN 978 0 85701 301 9

Printed and bound in Great Britain

Contents

FOREWORD

DAVID EMERSON[1]
DIRECTOR OF YOGA SERVICES,
THE TRAUMA CENTER, BROOKLINE, MA, USA

In April 2014, Dagmar Härle became one of the first ten people to be certified by my program at The Trauma Center in Brookline, MA, USA to teach Trauma-Sensitive Yoga (TSY) as an adjunctive clinical intervention for people with complex trauma, or what is also referred to in the literature as "treatment-resistant PTSD (post-traumatic stress disorder)." The TSY model that we developed at The Trauma Center is the first yoga-based intervention for complex trauma to receive federal funding for a randomized controlled trial. The results for the TSY cohorts, published in 2014, demonstrated a clinically significant reduction in PTSD symptomology as well as other intriguing findings (see van der Kolk *et al.* 2014).

Complex trauma is a framework for understanding the multi-layered impact that traumatic experiences, particularly interpersonal ones (that is, things that people do to each other, including physical and emotional abuse) have on individuals. At this point in time, thanks to the work of many researchers and clinicians, we have developed a good understanding of complex trauma; the time has now come to identify and promote good treatments. This book is an important step in that direction.

Myself and Dr Bessel van der Kolk, founder and Medical Director of The Trauma Center, started using TSY as a clinical intervention in 2003 in response to the growing understanding that trauma impacts the entire organism and that it is not just a disorder of thinking and behaving; in other words, treatments needed to respond to the whole

---

1   David Emerson is author of *Trauma-Sensitive Yoga in Therapy: Bringing the Body into Treatment* (W.W. Norton & Co., 2015).

person more effectively, and not just the part of a person that thinks about the past and plans for the future. In particular, we were interested in supporting the *person as they are*, right in front of us, in the present moment, which means, fundamentally, we are dealing with an *embodied being*. This seems rather obvious, to say that a person has a body, but it is arguable that mainstream therapy based on a psychodynamic or psychoanalytic conceptualization of a person practically ignores this fact; most therapists are dealing almost exclusively with the part of a person that can talk—it is truly a head game. In fact, the part of a person that thinks about the past, plans for the future, and talks about it is limited to a region of the brain called the frontal lobe or the neocortex—it is a very small part of a human organism. Granted, a lot of important things happen in that roughly one pound of gray matter, but, as Dagmar Härle points out in in this book, if we only attempt to treat this small part of a complexly traumatized person, we may end up being ineffective—letting down our clients and feeling defeated as caregivers. Without disregarding the valid need that many people have to process their traumatic experiences, to be heard and understood by another person (in some cases, a good therapist), TSY is an attempt to bring more of the person into the treatment paradigm: that which exists from the neck down. Importantly, and with not a small dose of irony, current research suggests that working with the *body* can have a positive effect on parts of the *brain* that are impacted by trauma, thereby connecting the brain and body, which, in the end, may prove to be the most important task of trauma treatment.

Along with an honest investigation of the true nature of traumatic experiences and the impact that these experiences have on the entire human organism, Dagmar Härle's book offers an interpretation of how a certain modified approach to yoga can be an important part of trauma treatment. Bringing together her expertise both as a clinician and as a yoga teacher, Dagmar navigates the connections between these two seemingly disparate but in actuality kindred domains so that readers can add a new dimension both to how they understand and how they treat trauma. It must be said, however, that not just any yoga will suffice. At The Trauma Center we spent years modifying yoga as commonly practiced in health clubs and yoga studios by millions of people around the world, and studying our modifications in clinical trials to produce what is now our model of TSY. In this book, Dagmar is careful to explain that in order to be used in trauma therapy, yoga must be modified, because if it is not, there is the very real danger that it may become another condition for reinforcing traumatic paradigms.

With her book, Dagmar Härle does the important work of calling attention to the growing understanding that trauma is an *organism-wide event* and not one limited to an individual's processes of thinking, behaving, and talking, but then she goes one step further, which is what makes this book a special contribution to the field—she offers practical, tangible tools that can be used by readers to treat trauma more effectively.

Acknowledgments

This book would not have been published without the enthusiastic support of a number of people. I would like to thank all of my teachers who shared their knowledge with me, as well as the pioneers who courageously took new paths and researched yoga in trauma therapy, for making it possible for me to even write this book. I am also grateful to my clients for their willingness to open up to something new. With their recognition, they have repeatedly emphasized the value of my work, and encouraged me to continue researching and ultimately put my experiences on paper. I would especially like to thank Iris Glanzmann for giving me important food for thought with her specific feedback on the effects of yoga in trauma therapy.

I thank Peter Streb for his valuable professional tips, as well as for his personal efforts, which contributed much to the creation of this book. Much credit is also due to David Emerson and Jenn Turner, the teachers who introduced me to Trauma-Sensitive Yoga (TSY) and allowed me to participate in their rich experiences. I would like to thank Inga Störkel, Andrea Szekeres, Erika von Arx, and Ursula Bubendorf—all of whom took the time to read the manuscript and gave me strength through their trust.

I would also like to say a big "thank you" to Sabine Tröndle for the professional photos included in the book. She turned the photo shoot into an experience where I could completely forget the camera.

I very much appreciate the efforts of a good friend who made an essential contribution to the readability of this book with her strong linguistic sensitivity and experience with text flow and style. And I would like to express my heartfelt gratitude to my husband, who always believes in me, and who has helped me to overcome many obstacles, with his patience and his understanding.

A big thanks goes to my editor of the original German edition of this book, Heike Carstensen, for her constructive criticism, and resulting successful collaboration. She both surprised and motivated me with her willingness to give my idea for this book a chance at Junfermann Verlag publishing company. And a big thanks to Natalie Watson and Singing Dragon for making it possible for the book to be published in English.

INTRODUCTION

Since primeval times, people have tried to cope with the adversities of life. There have always been upsetting and traumatizing events, but the methods for confronting the consequences of these shocks have varied greatly. They range from shamanic rituals such as soul retrieval to physical forms of expression such as singing and dancing to cognitive and narrative forms.

Many of our contemporary therapeutic approaches in the West are based on cognitive considerations. However, traumatization is not just shown in a change of convictions. Due to the lasting stress response, it is also displayed in the somatic effects that affect posture, physical reactions, and bodily sensations—phenomena that were the focus of treatment at other times and by other cultures. Feelings of numbness and being separated from one's own body often alternate with strong, overwhelming reactions to triggers, and in many cases make an efficient therapeutic approach more difficult. This book addresses these problems and focuses on the physical effects and reactions. Instead of introducing a new method, I see body-oriented work as a basis and supplement to the tried and tested techniques of trauma treatment.

WHY I WORK WITH YOGA
IN TRAUMA THERAPY

The idea of integrating yoga *asanas* (postures), *pranayama* (breathing exercises), and mindfulness into trauma therapy arose while working with my clients. When I completed my training in Somatic Experiencing and received my Master's degree in Psychotraumatology, I was convinced that exposure therapy combined with a body-oriented approach is expedient in treating complex post-traumatic stress disorders (PTSDs). I am still convinced of this, although it has become apparent to me that progress is not possible with every client when using this approach. For some people with complex trauma, the exposure of traumatic contents was simply not tolerable—relating to their own bodies was so disturbing to them that it triggered a response of panic and dissociation.

As a trained yoga teacher and yoga practitioner for many years, I have experienced the merits of bodywork in relation to a pronounced body awareness, increased mindfulness, and relaxation in everyday life, and presence in the here and now. My personal experience, as well as the feedback from my yoga students, encouraged me to integrate yoga into trauma therapy. I made my first attempt at this with a small group of female clients by offering them gentle yoga that allowed much space for mindful sensing. Above all, it was hardly directive. This means that it was fine if someone didn't want to do something or wasn't capable of it.

It was fascinating to see the kind of progress that the participants of my Mindful Yoga course made in therapy. Only now did it seem like the participants had a body that they could "expect" something of. It was finally possible to work with them. A female client confirmed my observations: "The therapy has only started through the yoga. Before this, I wasn't even in my body and couldn't do anything at all." These kinds of success encouraged me to increasingly integrate yoga into trauma therapy, especially in the individual setting, and allowed me to respond more to individual needs. I began to weave the yoga *asanas* and *pranayama* into trauma therapy, to work out resources with clients, promote body perceptions, and make it possible for them to approach their own bodies in a gentle way.

My work underwent systemization, expansion, and deepening through the basic course and subsequent certification program in Trauma-Sensitive Yoga (TSY) that I completed with David Emerson and his team at The Trauma Center in the Justice Resource Institute, Brookline, MA, USA. Bessel van der Kolk and David Emerson, pioneers and masters in the field of integrating yoga into trauma work, developed this therapeutic use of yoga based on the current research results regarding trauma and PTSD, which also takes the latest brain research and attachment theory into consideration. The positive effect on PTSD symptoms, which is comparable with results from other methods of trauma therapy, has now been scientifically proven by a number of studies.

Since I primarily work in a one-to-one setting in my practice as a trauma therapist, my intention was to have my experiences and principles of TSY flow into individual therapy. This enabled me to not only instruct groups and individuals, but also to use TSY in trauma individual therapy. Through my many years of experience in incorporating *asanas, pranayama*, and mindfulness into body-oriented trauma therapy, and combined with the principles of TSY, I created a tool for trauma therapists. With its help, possibilities for individual affect and self-regulation can be developed. This form of body-oriented work is also suitable for building up and strengthening personal resources.

When we speak about trauma, we tend to focus not on the physical experiencing, but on the event, which means the *story* that is told. We use it to explain the symptoms as well as changes in the thinking, feeling, behavior, and actions of the affected person. However, a trauma consists not only of the brain's continuing memories in the form of pictures, smells, sounds, and affects. Above all, a trauma is an experience that has happened to the body and has been stored there. Consequently, a trauma is also the story of a body that is frozen at the point in time of an event or, in the case of severely traumatized people, in the time period of the tormenting occurrences. The body is stuck in a constantly repeating stress response.

On the physical level, this paralysis is reflected in movement, breath, and posture patterns. In danger situations, the affected person would like to take action and escape the paralysis, but their body fails them instead of getting them to safety. In everyday life and situations in which they would normally be able to relax, they feel anxious, hypervigilant, and nervous, or numb and paralyzed. These states often alternate. The person is trapped between arousal and shut-down, between too much and too little. The body is not the place where traumatized people feel good. A female client expressed it like this: "I'm here," and pointed to her head. "What's down there should take me from A to B. I don't want to be concerned with it. It irritates me that it makes demands of me."

Exposure therapies are designed for clients to remember these traumatic occurrences within a safe environment and to report on them to therapists. This approach does not work for severely traumatized people due to the fact that they are unable to tolerate the exposure. As they suffer from flashbacks and dissociation, they are in no way able to benefit from the therapy—sometimes this endeavor causes more harm than benefit. To counteract this, the therapy usually starts with a stabilization phase. For example, visualizations are practiced in which clients see something like a "safe place" or a "vault" in which they can lock away terrible memories. Efforts are also focused on building a trusting therapeutic relationship. However, safe places and feelings of trust are rare for severely traumatized people, and it is often not even possible to get beyond the stabilization phase. Although we work on a sustainable therapeutic relationship, we avoid everything related to the trauma for the sake of the relationship. When people have relationship and attachment traumas, the relationship remains a fragile structure despite the good will of both parties, since being close to another person may already trigger stress for the client.

INTERACTION BETWEEN BODY AND PSYCHE

When both the physical reactions and the relationship with other people become a trigger, the idea of a transitional space can be helpful. This is a space in which the focus is not on the trauma or the relationship with the therapist, but a place where something new can happen. Yoga and other movement-focused forms, as well as art and expressive therapeutic approaches, offer such spaces. Since all of the unbearable affects, impulses, and sensations are played out in the body, offering possibilities of physical expression within this space suggests itself.

In contrast to other cultures, the West does not have a tradition for modulating mental states through physical activity such as those that have been practiced from time immemorial in African cultures through dance, singing, and rhythm, or Eastern cultures through forms of movement such as tai chi or qi gong. Yet all of us have probably had the experience of being able to regulate our mental states through movement. Dancing, singing, and moving rhythmically have a direct effect on our emotional state. Sad songs and rhythms make us wistful, and cheerful tunes brighten our mood. However, we do not use this empirical knowledge in a systematic way. We are also not accustomed to getting relief in this manner, and this path is blocked more than ever in stressful situations.

In Western culture, we rely on conversation to process difficult experiences. This is also reflected in the classic therapeutic setting that does not attach much importance to the training of body experience. We normally sit more or less upright on chairs, which is a posture that demands little proprioceptive and kinesthetic information processing. In this posture, we require almost no body awareness, and miss out on the opportunity to use our body for affect regulation.

This primal knowledge about the interaction between body and psyche is called "embodiment" by the cognitive sciences. It could also be understood as incarnation or corporealization. Embodiment describes the simple fact that emotions are not only expressed in the body, but that the opposite is also true: Body postures and sensations also influence the psyche. Since the outer stimuli are always accompanied by a somatic reaction, it is only logical that these frightening physical reactions become triggers on their own, because they can't be controlled. The body ultimately becomes a dangerous place. A female client got to the heart of this in one sentence: "The enemy is not on the outside!"

We make use of these considerations when we integrate *asanas* and *pranayama* into trauma therapy. The bottom-up approach focuses on the body with its forms of expression and sensations or its insensitivity. The goal is to gently "defrost" the body that is frozen in the trauma by offering unaccustomed posture and movement patterns to clients. We also experiment by exploring and changing breath patterns and movements, and subsequently consider the effect of the respective changes. Concentration on physical aspects such as stretching or powerful activity of a muscle and the mindful observation of body reactions in the constant alternation between exertion and recuperation during the practice trains the interoceptive awareness and self-exploration. Its goal is to establish a mind that is capable of observing instead of allowing itself to be overwhelmed by feelings. This benefits traumatized clients in both everyday life and the exposure therapy, because they have learned to control their affects much better.

Yoga is also a gentle exposure that is controlled by the clients themselves. The body is not ignored, but instead, becomes the center of attention. During the practice, clients can perceive all of the somatosensory sensations, such as the feeling of stretching, exertion, numbness, and signs of arousal such as an elevated pulse or change in breath frequencies. We could say that they remain "outside" and take up an observer position. So they may discover that there are body regions that are okay, and this gives them a feeling of safety. Or they may notice that not everything is numb to the same degree and that there are differences. In this way, they learn to differentiate. All of this helps them in their affect regulation and impulse control, which represents a basic precondition for successful trauma therapy.

YOGA IN TRAUMA THERAPY: LEARNING TO FEEL SAFE IN ONE'S OWN BODY

There are various methods that train body perception. Yoga, with its focus on structured body and breathing exercises, as well as the associated training of mindfulness, is especially well suited here. In yoga, we assume various body postures in the *asana* practice. We have a choice between different *asanas*, some simple and gentle, others complex and strenuous, depending on the client's physical capabilities, the space available, and the objectives of the therapy. In performing the *asanas*, muscles are consciously used through stretching, tensing, and relaxing. This trains the proprioceptive and kinesthetic perception, which is often inadequately developed in trauma clients. In many cases, trauma clients have been proven to have reduced activity in the insula and cingulate cortex—which is where, among other things, body sensations are registered. As a result, a differentiated body image is impeded (Levine 2010). *Asanas* give clients new interoceptive information, and we can assume that this counteracts the reduced activity in the insula and cingulate cortex.

In addition, yoga is very much engaged with our ability to influence the breath, and therefore the autonomic nervous system. People do not usually perceive their breath. When they freeze in fright, this can promote a breath pattern that overstimulates the sympathetic nervous system and maintains high stress levels. Learning body perception and guidance of the breath are valuable steps in the direction of empowerment and control.

Through yoga's typical structured, foreseeable approach, we offer additional safety and control. Instead of being in a "vacuum," we get into a defined yoga position together. We explore, change, and hold it, becoming better acquainted with the body in the process. We sense a movement, a tension, or a stretch with increasing clarity. Over time, we will also become aware of how emotions, thoughts, or memories are physically expressed. The repetition of similar positions or breathing exercises takes away the fear of what is unexpected.

Yoga is also called "meditation in motion." However, it differs from the concepts of classic mindfulness meditation in the seated position in that assuming body postures or performing movements is easier for trauma clients than sensing the body or observing thoughts and emotions during static sitting. Due to their constant vigilance, these clients often only perceive tension or numbness in a quiet posture. This makes them feel that they are all the more at the mercy of their demons.

Yoga has another major advantage: The exercises have a time limit! Being traumatized means having no control over when something begins and when it ends. In the vortex of overwhelming feelings, the sense of time is disturbed and there is no possibility of influence in escaping or ending the horror. Yoga that is customized for clients gives them control over the start and length of the exercise. This is accompanied by regaining a feeling of empowerment over themselves, their body, and their surrounding world. Trauma clients have two significant experiences in this process. First, they decide whether and when something begins, and they determine when it ends. Second, something ends, for example, the feeling of stretching in the muscle is just temporary. The progressive ability to observe teaches clients that every sensation and emotion has an end (cf. Emerson and Hopper 2011), which helps them to remain in their body. It allows them to tolerate physical reactions and sensations, feelings, and thoughts without being overwhelmed.

There are unmistakable parallels with body-oriented methods such as Somatic Experiencing (Levine 2010)—in which the application of switching back and forth between sympathetic and parasympathetic activity in the form of physical sensations, images, and/or thoughts is an example of the main approach. Once we have found resources through this trauma-oriented yoga in the form of postures, movements, breath control, or breathing exercises, clients acquire something to counter the pull of the trauma when memories and sensations threaten to overwhelm them.

Switching back and forth between the pull of the trauma and somatic resources (movements, postures, breath, awareness) slows down this process. Before we work with traumatic memories, it is good to practice slowing down with clients (cf. Rothschild 2002). We do exactly the same thing in trauma-oriented yoga: We assume a posture and sense something like activity in the muscles, acceleration of the heartbeat, or change of the breath rhythm—that is, an activation of the sympathetic nervous system in the body. Afterwards, we allow ourselves the time to feel how the tension lessens, the breath and pulse calm down, and the silence spreads. We create space for relaxation. Through the structured instructions and exercises, we provide safety to the clients. Within this offer, it is possible for them to have new experiences. At the same time, a space for change opens up—a space of transition or possibilities—in which clients can adapt and change their posture so that it is right for them. Clients have the experience that they can *do* something.

While I do not use TSY with all of my clients, I have noticed that people with complex trauma—and this is the target group for which I have written this book—benefit greatly from the idea of a transitional space in which they are allowed to try things out, reject them, and attempt them anew. I do not consider yoga to be a cure-all or the sole therapy for complex PTSDs. Instead, I see the body-oriented therapy approach as the basis on which I can build exposure therapy. With TSY, a measure of affect regulation ability can be attained in advance to help clients gain a sense of control over their feelings and sensations. In the further course of the therapy, the yoga *asanas* and breath control (*pranayama*) remain important resources, and can create a fruitful interaction of the body-oriented and cognitive focus.

ABOUT THIS BOOK

In the interest of readability and linguistic simplicity, I have decided to use the plural form for terms that relate to the therapist and the client, since they refer equally to women and men.

This book opens a space in which the traditional Indian concepts of yoga (the East) meet the modern insights of psychotraumatology and body-oriented therapy (the West). In order to do justice to both sides, I have organized this book in the following way.

Part I gives precedence to the West by briefly introducing the topics of trauma, post-traumatic stress disorder (PTSD), development and attachment trauma, and the customary treatment concepts.

Part II provides an introduction into the world of yoga with a brief summary of its historical development, philosophy, and an overview of its most important elements.

Current research in the areas of yoga with regard to health, stress, and PTSD are found in Part III. The form in which the yoga *asanas* and *pranayama* can be integrated into trauma therapy and what basic requirements are necessary for this purpose are explained in Part IV.

Part V is dedicated entirely to practice, and offers instructions for *asanas, pranayama*, and mindfulness. In Part VI, I link the therapeutic experience with the application of the yoga positions within the therapeutic context.

So I invite you to accompany me in this space of possibilities and encounter yourself, your interoceptive sensations, and your body perceptions as the first step. Without taking these into consideration, trauma-oriented yoga is not possible. This book is aimed at therapists working with clients who suffer from complex trauma, as well as laypeople and those affected by trauma who are interested in a body-oriented approach to the treatment of PTSDs.

Please note that any names mentioned in this book have been anonymized.

PART I

WEST: PSYCHO-TRAUMATOLOGY

1

THE EVENT

The term "trauma" is overused in the media. An entire city is traumatized from a shooting rampage at a school; people are traumatized after losing their job; a travel group is traumatized after a bus accident. However, a trauma should not be equated with a crisis or a general shock due to a serious event. A traumatizing situation impacts people on a profoundly personal level and shakes them to their innermost core. In the diagnostic manuals (the *International Statistical Classification of Diseases and Related Health Problems*, 10th revision, ICD-10, and *Diagnostic and Statistical Manual of Mental Disorders*, 5th edition, DSM-5[1]), we find two definitions that attempt to do justice to the severity of the events, as well as the reactions of the affected persons, in just a few words:

> A trauma is defined as an event or experience (of either brief or long duration) of an exceptionally threatening or catastrophic nature, which is likely to cause pervasive distress in almost everyone. (ICD-10)

The American DSM-IV (*Diagnostic and Statistical Manual of Mental Disorders*, 4th edn) describes trauma(s) as follows: An event or events that include a confrontation with actual or threatened death or serious injury or danger for one's own or others' physical integrity (cf. APA 2000; Graubner 2012; Lueger-Schuster 2008; Sass, Wittchen, and Zaudig 2003).

The DSM-5, published in 2013, describes the criteria like this: A person was subjected to the following events: death, death threat, real or threatened serious injury, real or threatened sexual violence. These events can either be seen as a potential trigger for PTSD due to direct

---

1   See http://apps.who.int/classifications/icd10/browse/2016/en and www.dsm5. org/psychiatrists/practice/dsm

exposure, being a witness, or indirectly when a close friend or relative has experienced something like this. Events that are connected with real or threatened death must have the character of an act of violence or an accident. In addition, the stressors include the repeated or extreme indirect experiencing of horrible details, often within the scope of the occupation. All of these criteria apply to adults. The DSM-5 also introduced a subtype for PTSD in children under the age of six years (US Department of Veterans Affairs no date).

Anyone can imagine themselves in an extremely threatening situation. If you do this for a moment, you will certainly sense that this is primarily a physical experience. Feel how you hold your breath and seize up. On an emotional level, the main responses are fear, panic, and anger, or even powerlessness, helplessness, or disgust. In an intense panic, thinking stops, the heartbeat slows down, the body becomes numb and limp, and you feel close to a state of faint or may actually become unconscious.

It is obvious that not every person will feel each event to be traumatizing in the same way. Due to the physical circumstances, the effect of having an experience of catastrophic magnitude is already different for children from what it is for adults. Women will experience it differently from men. There is also a difference as to whether a trauma is caused by human beings, an accident, or natural disaster, as well as how long the affected person was subjected to the traumatizing situation.

The number of traumas, as well as the support and closeness to other people after the event, also play just as much of a role in development of symptoms. In addition to the initial intensity of the symptoms, personal risk factors such as age (young or old), dissociation during the event(s), events in the personal history such as early separation and losses, insufficient social support, lower socio-economic status, and pre-existing conditions such as depression play an essential role. Examples of trauma-related factors are: intensity of the threat, repetitive traumas, intentional actions by the perpetrator, irreversible harm through the trauma, as well as feelings of shame and guilt. This is why the concept of trauma requires further differentiation.

DIFFERENTIATION OF THE TERM "TRAUMA"

A one-time traumatic experience is classified as a *Type I* trauma, and a persistent traumatization is called a *Type II* trauma. The complex traumatization or Type II trauma is differentiated according to its duration, degree of severity, and its effects on the Type I traumatization personality.

Judith Herman summarizes complex traumatization as follows:

> The client was subjected over a prolonged period to totalitarian control. Examples include hostages, prisoners of war, concentration camp survivors, and survivors of some religious cults. This also includes those subjected to totalitarian systems in sexual and domestic life, including those subjected to domestic battering, childhood physical or sexual abuse, and organized sexual exploitation. (2003, p.167f.)

Within this context, the term "allostatic load" is also used, which is the cumulative physiological "cost" of an ongoing stress situation (see Glover 2006).

Even though the consequences of traumatic events have been known for many years, the effect of a one-time traumatization on personality and sense of self is hard to compare with the impairments that result from a lengthy trauma experience. This means that the diagnosis of post-traumatic stress disorder (PTSD) is not completely accurate for the last-mentioned group of victims (those victims of organized sexual exploitation) since they frequently display much more complex symptoms (Herman 2003). This is called an attachment (or bonding) trauma or developmental trauma (Maercker 2009), when the triggering experience occurred very early in life.

The sense of life-threatening danger is something completely different for a child, especially when the threat comes from a caregiver. If a child or adolescent experiences episodes of physical mistreatment, sexual assault, or physical neglect, as well as a multitude of cumulative microtraumas through ongoing debasement, excessive demands, lacking a sense of emotional security, emotional abuse or neglect, or has suffered from multiples cases of separation or loss, the resulting damage and accompanying disorders of personality development are much more extensive. A child who must live in the confusing environment where the caregiver(s) is (are) simultaneously the perpetrator(s) is therefore forced to protect the attachment relationship (Schreiber-Willnow and Hertel 2006). A male client expressed this as follows: "After all, I somehow had to get along with him [his father]. If I no longer felt anything, I could do what he demanded of me. Then I was safer."

Many authors advocate introducing the term of "developmental trauma," since the complexity of the symptoms cannot be explained comprehensively enough with the term "post-traumatic stress disorder," and because the classic methods of treating PTSD fall short in these cases (D'Andrea *et al.* 2012; Ford *et al.* 2013; Kisiel *et al.* 2014; Stolbach 2007; van der Kolk 2005).

In summary, a traumatic situation shocks people in their entire being—their thoughts, feelings, and physical reactions. It is often overlooked that the body, even if it doesn't display any outer injuries, has suffered a life-threatening situation, and the physiological reactions remain in the memory. In addition to all of the other sensory impressions, the affected person is just as unlikely to forget the sensation of numbness and helplessness. The same applies to their inability to simply shake off the memory of the racing heart or nausea during the traumatic incident. In order to deal with these tormenting sensations, they develop patterns of physical reactions that include a change in breathing habits or posture and movement tendencies. These habituated body programs make a considerable contribution toward maintaining emotions and thoughts in a vicious circle.

2

THE IMPACT

POST-TRAUMATIC STRESS DISORDER (PTSD)

It was only recognized in the second half of the eighteenth century that fear and terror have effects on the psyche. With terms such as "general nervous shock" and "traumatic neurosis," Herbert W. Page (1845–1926) and Emil Kraepelin (1856–1926) made a considerable contribution to these correlations being taken seriously. In both the First and Second World Wars, it became apparent that soldiers reacted to the experiences of battle and war with various symptoms described as shell shock, battle neurosis, or combat fatigue. However, the opinion at the time was that only "inferior" and "useless" people were afflicted by such symptoms. It wasn't until the Vietnam War that a more realistic and differentiated perspective gained support, which helped psychotraumatology make its breakthrough. People slowly had to accept that not only those with a "weak" nature reacted to horrible events with psychological symptoms, but that the same also applied to individuals who were psychologically healthy and stable (cf. Maercker 2009).

It could also no longer be overlooked that other extreme experiences, such as sexual violence, torture, or accidents, led to similar reactions. In the 1970s, studies investigating the basal cognitive processes of dealing with traumatic stress had pointed out a symptom pattern that is typical for PTSD: intrusions, avoidance, and feelings of guilt (cf. Maercker 2009). In 1980, PTSD was included in the American DSM for the first time. In the ICD and DSM classification systems, the current definition reflects the symptoms of intrusions and avoidance observed by Horowitz in 1974. The list was further expanded with hyperarousal (increased psychophysiological level of agitation and overexcitation), as well as by a time factor (symptoms last longer than one month).

SYMPTOMS OF POST-TRAUMATIC STRESS DISORDER

Let's take a closer look at the PTSD symptom triad of intrusions, avoidance, and hyperarousal.

Intrusions are displayed through pictures, sounds, or other vivid impressions of the traumatic occurrence that intrude into the affected person's sleep. They manifest in the form of recurring dreams or nightmares or as very realistic, detailed flashbacks that catapult the affected person from the present into the past and into this traumatic event.

However, the intrusive perceptions include not only pictures or vivid impressions, but also physical sensations that play out in the body as if they are happening in the here and now and have an intrusive character. Even though it may feel good to us to stretch our arm muscles when reaching upward above our head, this may become a somatosensoric trigger[1] for victims of torture, reminding them of the past and of their tormentors.

Hyperarousal is exhibited in physical reactions. As if out of nowhere, the breath falters and the body stiffens. The heart skips a beat just to pound even harder after that. Clients may suffer from somatoform dissociation phenomena such as inexplicable physical sensations or body reactions and symptoms, as well as from somatosensory memories and/or flashback-like physical sensations that arise during traumatic memories. In many cases, these physical symptoms are associated with shame and are therefore kept secret, or the clients have multiple attempts at clarification behind them without establishing a medical finding.

Moreover, a trauma can lower the arousal threshold of the autonomic nervous system. This means that strains have an earlier, longer-lasting effect, and even minor stress stimuli can lead to a more intense state of arousal. Hyperarousal can be displayed in the form of trouble getting to sleep and staying asleep, as well as in hypervigilance, the inability to relax, and jumpiness (cf. Maercker 2009).

---

1   Somatosensory (Greek *soma* "body"; Latin *sensorius* "serving the sensation") means "related to the physical sensitivity." In the somatosensory cortex, the information of the skin receptors that receive the environmental stimuli (exteroception) and the receptors inside the body, i.e. self-awareness (proprioception), are processed in the somatosensory cortex. The somatosensory perception therefore applies to the proprioceptive (organs, muscles, and joints) and tactile (skin) sensations.

The affected person uses every means possible to *avoid* trauma triggers such as thoughts, activities, places, and people—as well as physical sensations—that remind them of the traumatic occurrence. Clients report that they feel emotionally numb and alienated (*numbing*). This flattening of the emotional world and a continuing sense of general alienation is related not only to their personal and social environment; it also applies to their own body, which feels completely or partially numb. Many clients are not even aware of this numbness because they have become accustomed to it.

COMPLEX POST-TRAUMATIC STRESS DISORDER, ATTACHMENT TRAUMA, AND DEVELOPMENTAL TRAUMA

A diagnosis of complex PTSD is given when the clinical picture goes beyond the above-mentioned classic PTSD group of symptoms. For example, this could include affect regulation disorders, depressive symptoms, anxiety disorders and panic attacks, attachment disorders with intense mistrust or insufficient self-protection, insufficient self-care, the victimization of others, or acting like a victim (cf. Maercker 2009).

Attachment trauma and developmental trauma leave even more profound traces in people's lives. The younger the affected person was at the time of the traumatizing experience, the more severe the consequences. If the sensations and feelings are not calmed from the outside by a caregiver—if this person does not appropriately respond to the child's needs—the immature brain is flooded by the release of stress hormones, which impairs the child's development. "Complex post-traumatic stress disorders are always also attachment disorders..." (Wöller 2006, p.40).

It is not just the point in time of the emotional shock, but the destruction of the basic trust in the person from whom the child expects protection that is the most serious moment for child development (Steele 1994). This means that the influence of interactive experiences between children and their primary caregiver plays an even more important role than the traumatic events (Stern 1985). If we want to understand people with complex trauma, attachment theory, developed by Mary Ainsworth in the 1970s, is helpful. She subdivided the behavior of one-year-old children in the Strange Situation (brief separation from the mother) into the attachment categories of secure, insecure-ambivalent, insecure-avoidant, and disorganized (see Grossmann 2011).

For securely attached children, the caregiver fulfills the role of the "safe haven," always offering protection to the child when needed. Insecure-ambivalent and insecure-avoidant children are not able to trust in their attachment person's availability. The only way out of the oppressive and threatening situation is to avoid the relationship. Insecurely-ambivalently attached children show that they are fearful and dependent on their attachment person since the behavior of the latter is neither predictable nor comprehensible. The constant alternation between approachable and unapproachable behavior leads to the necessity of the child's attachment system constantly being activated. These children cannot develop any positive expectations, because the attachment person does not offer any reliable protection— even when they are nearby.

Traumatized children more frequently display one of the two insecure attachment patterns. A further attachment pattern of disorganized attachment is primarily associated with neglect and abuse. These children suffer from the fact that the person who should guarantee their protection represents a threat or they suffer from the consequences of their own psychotrauma. If the traumatizing caregiver displays frightening-terrifying or a fearful-terrified behavior, children are unable to develop a uniform attachment strategy for attaining protection and comfort. They behave in an avoidant-disorganized or clinging-disorganized way that is shown by how they search for closeness and then behave with aggression or resistance in the same breath.

When children must protect themselves against the person from whom they obviously need protection, they find themselves in a hopeless situation. They are unable to develop successful strategies for coming into contact with their closest caregiver. Consequently, they remain stuck in an approaching–avoiding conflict. This relationship behavior is also apparent in their adult lives, and becomes visible in therapy as well (cf. Wöller 2006).

ATTACHMENT TRAUMAS AND THEIR EFFECTS

Children who grow up with caregivers incapable of attunement—adults who also cannot reflect or regulate their own emotional states—are in a constant state of stress. Relationships with these caregivers are frequently broken off and not re-established for a long time afterward.

If the break is not mended, these children stay alone in their dysregulated state with its profound negative affects for too long and for too often. The cortisol level and other stress hormones may be continuously elevated, which has serious and long-term effects on their ability to regulate stress. Since the traumatizing parental (caregiving) figures are incapable of "repairing" the interruption of the attachment relationship through calming and comforting behavior, it is these experiences that trigger fear and insecurity in the children when they enter into close intimate relationships as adults—despite their longing to have them. The concern that their own misconduct will lead to an irreparable break causes them to either become overly conforming in order to not endanger the attachment, or they destroy every arising situation of intimacy on their own (cf. Wöller 2006).

The psychoanalyst Allan N. Schore, who studies the problems of the distress system from the perspective of attachment research, points out two forms of relationship trauma: abuse and neglect. Abuse, which can also be called mistreatment, results in an over-stimulation, a hyperarousal, and activates the sympathetic nervous system. Neglect can lead to an under-stimulation that is controlled by the parasympathetic nervous system. Too much or too little—both are unbearable. The most serious effect of early traumatization through abuse and neglect is the loss and/or insufficient ability to regulate one's own feelings. This creates a habitual tendency to let oneself fall into primitive, parasympathetic states—which is typical for a regulation system that is immature in terms of its development (Schore, quoted in Sachsse and Roth 2008).

In summary, this means that we must have therapeutic instruments available that help clients to improve their affect regulation and prevent them from dissociating, suffering flashbacks, etc., and/or falling into the parasympathetic state of atony. At the same time, we need a form of relationship that is as different as possible from the relationship patterns learned through earlier traumatic relationships.

ADVERSE CHILDHOOD EXPERIENCE (ACE)

The large-scale Adverse Childhood Experience (ACE) study is concerned with the complex effects of traumas in childhood. The Centers for Disease Control and Prevention in Atlanta and Kaiser Permanente in San Diego studied more than 17,000 adults. Ten different types of childhood traumas were analyzed—three types of abuse, two forms of neglect, and five types of dysfunctional family structures. The results show a clear connection between ACE and chronic physical and psychological diseases, as well as their effects in adulthood. Examples of this are lung and respiratory diseases, hepatitis, depression, and suicidal tendencies. Multiple ACEs indicate a premature death of the affected person, who passes away an average of 20 years earlier than those without ACEs. There is apparently a correlation between ACE and social, emotional, and cognitive impairments. This is reflected in health behavior and is frequently accompanied by social problems, which ultimately means a shorter life expectancy in the final analysis. The ACE study clearly proves that we are not "just" dealing with PTSD symptoms in the work with complex PTSDs, but also with diverse clinical pictures since the vulnerable childhood years make people extremely susceptible to far-reaching disorders (Felitti and Anda 1997; Newlin, 2011).

A sequential traumatization in adulthood can also lead to a destruction of personality, self-image, sense of wellbeing, and health in the long term. The following table shows an overview of the simple PTSD symptoms, the symptom fields of a complex PTSD, developmental trauma, and the consequences of ACEs.

The symptoms and symptom fields of a simple PTSD, a complex PTSD, a developmental trauma, and Adverse Childhood Experience (ACE)

Symptoms of a simple PTSD according to DSM-5 (APA 2013)	Symptom fields of a complex PTSD (Herman 2003)	Symptom fields of developmental traumatization (according to van der Kolk 2009)
A. Confrontation with a traumatic event: Death, death threat, real or threatened serious injury, real or threatened sexual violence, either as direct exposure, through witnessing, or indirectly (close people affected). Events that are connected with real or threatened death must have the character of an act of violence or accident. Repeated or extreme indirect experiencing of horrible details, often within the scope of an occupation. All of these criteria apply to adults	Disorders of affect regulation: • Persistent dysphoria • Chronic suicidal preoccupation • Self-injury • Explosive or suppressed anger (may alternate) • Compulsive or extremely inhibited sexuality	Exposure: • Frequent or chronic exposure to one or various development-inhibiting interpersonal traumatizations (i.e. being deserted, betrayal of trust; physical, emotional, or sexual abuse or encroachments) • Subjective experience of anger, betrayal of trust, fear, resignation, humiliation, or shame

B. Intrusions:
 	
1. Recurring and powerful distressing memories (pictures, thoughts, and perceptions)
2. Recurrence of distressing dreams
3. Dissociation reactions such as flashbacks
4. Intensive stress after exposure of trauma triggers
5. Physiological reactivity after exposure
	Disorders of perception and consciousness:
	
	• Amnesia or hyperamnesia related to the traumatic events
	• Occasional dissociation phases
	• Depersonalization/derealization
	• Recurrence of traumatic event as intrusive symptoms or through constant brooding
		Triggered patterns:
		
		• Dysregulation in presence of stimuli, i.e. high or low stimuli response. Changes persist and do not return to baseline; they are not reduced in their intensity by becoming aware of them
		  • Affective
		  • Somatic
		• Behavior of reenactment; self-injury
		• In relationships, e.g. through clinging, defiant behavior, mistrust, and deference
		• Self-hatred and self-accusation

cont.

Symptoms of a simple PTSD according to DSM-5 (APA 2013)	Symptom fields of a complex PTSD (Herman 2003)	Symptom fields of developmental traumatization (according to van der Kolk 2009)
C. Avoidance: 1. Conscious avoidance of trauma-related stimuli 2. Conscious avoidance of activities, places, and people who awaken memories D. Negative changes in relation to perception and moods: 1. Inability to remember an important aspect of the trauma 2. Persistent negative beliefs and expectations about oneself or the world 3. Persistent recriminations (against oneself or others) in relation to the trauma 4. Persistent negative feelings (fear, horror, annoyance, guilt, and/or shame) 5. Distinctly diminished interest or reduced participation in important activities 6. Feeling of being detached or alienated from others 7. Restricted range of the affect	Disturbed self-perception: • Feelings of helplessness and paralysis of any type of initiative • Feelings of shame and guilt, self-incrimination • Feelings of being dirty and stigmatized • Feeling of being basically different from others	Persistent changed attributions and expectations: • Negative self-attributions • Mistrust toward protective caregivers • Loss of expectations to be protected by others (people and institutions) • Loss of the belief in social justice/retaliation • Victim role
E. Persistent symptoms of elevated arousal: 1. Irritability or outbursts of rage 2. Autoaggression or inconsideration 3. Hypervigilance (extreme alertness) 4. Exaggerated fright reactions 5. Difficulties in concentration 6. Sleep disorders	Disturbed perception of perpetrator: • Constantly thinking about the perpetrator • Unrealistic assessment of perpetrator (omnipotent, idealization, or thankfulness) • Feelings of a special or supernatural relationship • Assumption of perpetrator's value system	Functional impairments: • Upbringing/education • Family • In contact with same-aged people • Legal • Professional

F. The clinical picture lasts longer than one month G. Effect on functional capability significant symptom-related stress or functional restrictions	Relationship problems: • Isolation and retreat • Disorders in intimate relationships • Search for a rescuer • Persistent mistrust • Inability to protect self
H. Exclusion: Symptoms are not produced by medications, substance abuse, or illness Must be specified when dissociative symptoms exist: • Depersonalization • Derealization	Changes in value system: • Loss of firm beliefs • Feelings of hopelessness and desperation

ACE (Adverse Childhood Experience) (Felitti and Anda 1997)

ACE leads to massively increased health risks in various areas of health. These include:

- Alcohol abuse
- Drug consumption
- Depression
- Suicide
- Smoking
- More than 50 sexual partners
- Sexually transmittable diseases
- Physical inactivity
- Being severely overweight
- Ischemic heart disease

The table makes it clear at a glance that the effects are clearly differentiated from each other. As a result, the treatment must be attuned to each of the clinical pictures.

Clients frequently do not seek treatment as a result of PTSD symptoms. The correlation between the unclear symptom picture and a traumatization can often not be recognized by both, the affected person and the therapist. "Classic" PTSD symptoms such as flashbacks, intrusions, and hyperarousal are often masked by avoidance behavior that has been perfected over decades to escape the intolerable intrusions and arousals. Avoidance is also frequently not perceived as such by clients, and is only talked about when very precise questions are asked. The entire life of the client is consciously or unconsciously centered on provoking as few triggers as possible.

The restrictions in everyday life are incisive and have an effect on academic performance, education, career choices, and professional success, as well as on personal relationships and health behavior. These difficulties are based on the extreme feelings of powerlessness and helplessness during the traumatization. The affected persons dissociate due to the overwhelming occurrence, which leads to habitual dissociation. As a consequence of this, they quickly feel overwhelmed, helpless, and powerless. They panic or become angry and enraged. However, the typical hyperarousal symptoms are not present. A habitual dissociation is also expressed in the physical experiencing—a feeling of weakness, paralysis, dizziness, and being on the verge of fainting. At such moments, the affected person is no longer capable of speaking. Their body goes limp, and their hands become cold and moist. These "physical flashbacks" intensify the panic because clients have nothing to counteract them with. According to one client, "The feeling of not being able to move and fight the helplessness is an absolute horror."

These interoceptively perceived physical sensations in particular dig their way deeply into the memory of the clients, and lead to an increasing fear of "being abandoned by one's own body." The experience of "my body doesn't get me to safety!" is far-reaching.

DISSOCIATION

Like intrusions, avoidance, and hyperarousal, dissociation can be the result of a traumatic event. If dissociation occurs during the traumatic event, this has a decisive effect on the severity of the symptoms. If there is even just a tiny remnant of self-empowerment, the consequences of a traumatization are often less pronounced than for complete dissociation and immobility, with feelings of powerlessness and helplessness during the event.

On the physical level, dissociation and the accompanying immobility can even make sense. As long as people are able to sense pain or anger and see a possibility for taking action, they will instinctively attempt to get away from the threatening danger. Yet, immobility in particular was an important evolutionary survival factor. The state of shut-down or defeat (giving up) actually protects against movements that could worsen the injuries or incite the perpetrator's aggression. No longer being able to move, being cut off from feelings, and dissociating can also be understood as the organism's defense strategy that ensures survival.

There is a difference between tonic and flaccid immobility. In tonic immobility, an explosive flight response in connection with aggressive behavior is still possible. Feelings such as anger or rage are still present in this state, but are suppressed. If it looks like this active defense is not going to work, the organism transitions into "flaccid immobility," controlled by the parasympathetic nervous system. In this state, both the emotional involvement and any type of disposition to take action disappear. Those who end up with parasympathetic dominance during the trauma will tend to display dissociative reactions due to the conditioning of the trauma-related trigger. On the other hand, those who end up with a sympathetic reaction will tend to feel rage or fear. As the last degree of the scale, fainting appears to be closely associated with disgust when bodily fluids such as blood or sperm are involved (Schauer and Elbert 2010).

The probability that dissociative moments occurred in attachment or developmental traumas is very high—a child's organism will "give up" due to just its physical inferiority since resistance can easily be overcome and/or overlooked.

SOMATOFORM DISSOCIATION

In addition to the above-listed symptoms, some clients exhibit somatoform symptoms such as pain in their sexual organs, occasional sensorial malfunctions, or hypersensitivity or insensitivity to pain. At the same time, the classic PTSD criteria of intrusion and avoidance behavior are missing. Nijenhuis *et al.* (1996, 2004) have described the clinical picture of somatoform dissociation. As shown by various studies of risk groups, the correlation between the number of experienced traumas and the extent of somatoform dissociation is high, especially for early Type II traumatizations (see also Nijenhuis 2009).

The symptoms of somatoform dissociation include the so-called negative attributes such as anesthesia, with occasional loss of sensitivity, analgesia, an occasional loss of pain sensation, and loss of motoric control such as movements, the voice, swallowing, etc. Examples of so-called positive dissociative symptoms are somatoform components of non-conscious processes such as the histrionic phenomena and attacks, fixed ideas, reactivated traumatic memories (i.e. localized psychogenic pain), as well as dissociative movement sequences.

Clients experiencing somatoform dissociation phenomena will either seek medical help because the unbearable pain or loss of motor control indicates a physical cause, or they will simply ignore them. This may include sensations of numbness, the complete loss of physical sensations, or insensitivity to pain. As in the co-morbid disorders of PTSD, the correlation between somatoform dissociation symptoms and traumatization is not easy to recognize.

For assessing the symptom severity of the somatoform phenomena, SDQ-5 or SDQ-20 (Somatoform Dissociation Questionnaire, versions with 5 or 20 items; see Nijenhuis 2009) are suitable. This questionnaire frequently opens up the conversation about correlations between trauma, the body, and physical sensations, or the lack thereof. It delivers good arguments for a body-related therapeutic approach, which does not make sense to many clients at first glance.

3

WHY DOESN'T IT STOP WHEN IT'S OVER?

This question is more than justified. In cognitive terms, the affected person has long understood that the trauma is over, yet it still appears that they are prohibited from leading a normal, or perhaps even happy life.

The causes don't just lie in flawed thinking and searching for the structures that are responsible for it, because the processing of information during trauma doesn't happen in the cerebrum. The instinctive actions, drive for survival, and patterns of action required for this process fall under the responsibilities of the phylogenetically older "lower" regions of the brain. This is why we should first take a look at how information is processed in the brain.

The limbic brain structures of the amygdala and the hippocampus play a key role here. When the issue is survival, there is no time for reflection. As a result, the order of the survival patterns must be established instinctively.

THE HIERARCHY OF INFORMATION PROCESSING

A potentially traumatic event that causes stress is followed by the biologically established stress–response cascade (see also the figure below):

1. Freeze—startle reaction—orienting response

2. Fight/flight—sympathetic activation, body is ready for action

3. Fright—panic, tonic immobility, dissociation starts

4. Flag—flaccid immobility, parasympathetic activation, dissociation grows

5. Faint—loss of consciousness

In the first heart-stopping moment, the body briefly freezes and tries
to grasp the situation in order to coordinate the appropriate reaction to
it. If the situation is perceived as threatening, the sympathetic nervous
system is activated on the second and third stage of the cascade. People
feel slightly dizzy, the heartbeat accelerates, the mouth becomes dry,
the muscles tense, and a feeling of numbness and irreality arises. The
body is in uproar and equipped for flight or fight.

The fourth stage of the scale—tonic immobility—causes
tachycardia, constriction of blood vessels, hypertension, and
hyperalertness. Aggression is inhibited, and the fear becomes
overwhelming. Both fight and flight are still possible, should these
individuals see an opportunity for rescue. The onset of immobility
is faster in this stage and also ends more quickly than in the state of
flaccid immobility. Dissociative phenomena increase.

In the fifth stage of the scale, the individual goes limp and
surrenders. The blood pressure falls, the blood vessels expand, the
heartbeat slows down, all emotional feelings are numbed, and both
thinking and the sensations of pain are shut down. In this state of
physical and emotional anesthesia, the individual dissociates—which
means that they are no longer present in the outer world. The cause
of this is the activation of the parasympathetic nervous system. The
situation signals helplessness and hopelessness. Fight or flight appears
to be impossible and/or futile (Putnam 1997). At this stage, the
immobility starts slowly and stops just as slowly.

The sixth and last stage of the cascade leads to faint (cf. Schauer
and Elbert 2010). In this situation, the amygdala is active. Its function
includes the evaluation of incoming information on an emotional
level—it is responsible for affective states that are associated with
threat and danger. It stores information in the form of pictures and
physical sensations, which are located in the emotionally implicit
memory system, and it is frequently very difficult or not even possible
to access them with words, and also very difficult to erase.

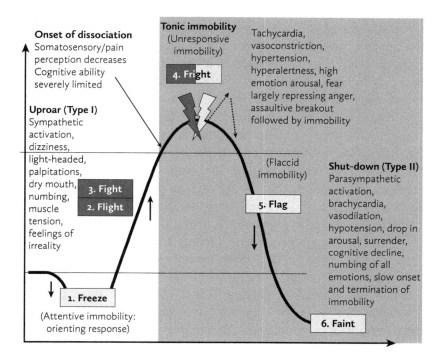

The left side (see the figure above) represents the PTSD type with sympathetic arousal (Type I). The right side, which shows the further course of the defense cascade, describes this occurrence in a complex traumatization (Type II).

Among other things, the "control center" of the brain—the thalamus or diencephalon—is responsible for transmitting relevant information from the body and the sensory organs to the cerebral cortex. In order for people to become aware of their sensitive–sensory information, all of the ascending pathways—with the exception of the olfactory pathway—must be interconnected in the thalamus before they continue on their way to the cortex. However, very little of the sensory information makes its way to the cortex in a state of major danger. The only exception here is odors. The well-known smelling bottle from times past that helped ladies get over their faints can still be used today to retrieve clients from a state of high arousal.

HOW EXPERIENCES ARE PROCESSED IN THE BRAIN

Information flows together from the various sensory systems in the hippocampus. This is processed and sent back to the cortex from here, which means that it plays a key role in consolidation of memory (conveyance of memory contents from the short-term to the long-term memory). In traumatic situations, the hippocampus is weakened. However, together with the prefrontal cortex, it is also responsible for putting the information evaluated by the amygdala into context. Moreover, it is responsible for the cognitive reconciliation with previous information that is transferred to an explicit and/or declarative memory.[1] The weakening of the hippocampus therefore causes a cessation of cognitive reconciliation.

The amygdala system assumes control, and incoming information is not transferred to the declarative memory. As a result, the contents of the traumatic memory are "stuck" in the implicit sensory memory (situationally accessible memory, SAM). They are only partially accessible through words and easy to trigger. Since they are not transferred to this declarative, autobiographical, verbally accessible memory (VAM), they also cannot be integrated into the life story (cf. dual representation theory; see Brewin, Dagleish and Joseph 1996).

Through the functional weakening of the hippocampus, the amygdala is unmodulated and the information processing remains unfiltered. Consequently, the stimuli are stored as sensory information according to their *emotional* significance. This leads to a fragmentation of the memory contents and an intrusive experiencing in the form of pictures, as well as other sensory memories. An inappropriate message of danger occurs, which results in an overly generalized fear response to the trauma trigger. The fear response stored in the amygdala can be easily triggered and cannot be erased. At best, it can only be inhibited. This inhibition occurs through the orbifrontal cortex, which works closely with the hippocampus (Grawe 2004).

So the affected person suffers from the consequences of memories. These are stored in the subcortical regions of the brain as a threat and triggered over and over again. This state is comparable with the situation of infants, who do not yet have any ability to modulate external stimuli. They are also easy to trigger and a caregiver is needed to help infants regulate their feelings.

---

1   The declarative memory can differentiate between the past and the present, and the information is linguistically and semantically available.

In traumatized people, an easily activated fright structure has been created that contains cognitive, emotional, sensory, and sensomotoric elements. Each time a trauma trigger is recalled, the entire cascade is initiated. This intensifies the conditioning. Clients therefore do everything to avoid the triggers. Since this also means that no new corrective experiences can be had, avoidance has the effect of just cementing the process.

> The higher (cortical) centers of the brain are viewed as responsible for abstraction, perception, reasoning, language, and learning. Sensory integration and intersensory association, in contrast, occur mainly within lower (subcortical) centers. Lower parts of the brain are conceptualized as developing and maturing before higher-level structures. Development and optimal functioning of higher-level structures are thought to be dependent, in part, on the development and optimal functioning of the lower-level structures. (Figley 2002, p.127, cited in Fisher, Murray and Bundy 1991)

In the treatment of PTSDs, the affected person's age at the time of the traumatization and the type of trauma experienced play a major role. Does a simple or complex traumatization affect an adult, a person who has resources, and whose brain structure is mature? Or are we dealing with a complex traumatization or neglect during childhood in which the affected person had neither the physical nor the cognitive resources and an immature brain structure at the time of the events? If it was not possible for the person to first learn affect modulation and regulation, the effects on personal development are devastating. Although an involuntarily easily triggered fear structure develops in the amygdala in both cases, it is much more difficult—and usually even impossible—to transfer this into consciously accessible, contextualized hippocampal memories in the case of traumatization in childhood. Yet it is absolutely necessary in both cases that, figuratively speaking, the amygdala must "comprehend" that the triggers from the past no longer represent a threat.

The limbic system primarily learns from experience. An inner map is formed that helps it to differentiate between situations and people that are safe, those that are still acceptable, or those that are dangerous. On the basis of their experiences, neglected or abused people react in a different emotional and physical way to their surrounding world. In order to explain the world to themselves, they have adopted a different way of thinking from those who have been spared these experiences.

HOW CAN TRAUMATIC EXPERIENCES BE INTEGRATED?

The integration of traumatic experiences must occur on the physical, emotional, and cognitive level:

1. In order to change the map of the limbic structures, traumatized people must be able to have new experiences that contradict the old, and that change their physical and emotional experiencing.

2. Trauma clients require support in order to separate from their harmful thought patterns and be able to replace them with positive or supportive beliefs.

3. For the successful treatment of traumatic experiences, it is essential that trauma memories are transferred into the explicit VAM. They should ideally be stored in the implicit procedural memory (SAM) and at best, but more deficiently, in the VAM. The after-effects of a PTSD can essentially be ascribed to a dissociation of the implicit and explicit trauma memory (see van der Kolk, Burbridge, and Suzuki 1997; van der Kolk, Fisler, and Blom 1996; Wessa and Flor 2002).

Let's first look at point 2. Cognitive therapy methods offer techniques of cognitive restructuring for dysfunctional thought patterns. They focus on the schemata changed by traumatization. In order to process a trauma, the affected person tries to bring this traumatic occurrence into harmony with their previous thought patterns. This results in dysfunctional programs such as: "That something this terrible happened to me can only mean that I deserved it/am worthless/am bad." Thoughts that are intended to keep the feelings of losing control at bay, such as "I can't ever trust anyone again," can be reinforced by the attempt to mentally get everything back into balance. Avoidance behavior, as well as thoughts and beliefs that disturb the cognitive restructuring and emotional processing, perpetuate the PTSD symptoms.

If we base this on the considerations of point 3, we can expect trauma clients to have a decrease in symptoms if it is possible to remove the dissociation of explicit and implicit trauma memory in the therapy. Through therapeutic measures—all of which ultimately include a re-experiencing and processing of the trauma-relevant stimuli in a secure environment—a fully developed explicit, verbally accessible trauma memory is established. As a result of this approach, the fear reaction of the amygdala is gradually inhibited ever more effectively. A repeated confrontation with the specific sensory stimuli and corresponding context information makes a contribution to this process. "The structure of the inhibition is not a matter of insight but a function of the frequency with which the fear-triggering stimuli and fear-inhibiting context can be simultaneously activated" (Grawe 2004, p.163).

We can also assume that trauma memories have been inadequately integrated into a context from time and space—from both the previous and subsequent information, as well as autobiographical memories. So the possibility of verbalization is hardly pronounced, and the resulting memory has neither a temporal context nor is it connected with the later information (e.g. "I'm still alive"). These facts produce the here-and-now feeling of intrusive memories (Ehlers 1999; Ehlers and Clark 2000). Only through working out a coherent narration of the event—which includes the context information as well as the trauma memories—the division of implicit and explicit memory can be removed.

COGNITIVE PROCESSING ON ITS OWN IS NOT ENOUGH

The cognitive processing and integration of traumatic events is absolutely necessary and part of a successful trauma therapy. There is no doubt that thought patterns represent a major strain and inhibit people from having a satisfactory life. However, solely focusing the therapeutic approach on the dysfunctional beliefs is not enough. This issue is precisely what causes many clients to be close to desperation, because they know very well that the overwhelming feelings do not have their cause in the present but in the past. Yet this perception in no way leads to an improvement of their wellbeing. The activation of the implicit memory contents with its trauma-relevant stimuli is also intolerable for some. This makes it virtually impossible to work out a coherent narration. Consequently, the talking cure—which helps the affected person succeed in thinking differently and/or having a coherent narration—is only one part of the solution.

If we take the hierarchy of information processing in the therapeutic process into consideration, the affected person initially needs help with affect regulation. Once this succeeds, the traumatic event can be addressed, which makes it possible to also work through trauma-related, dysfunctional thought patterns and to replace them with functional ones.

In order to access traumatic memory contents, therapists must have tools available that also reach the subcortical brain structures. It has already been shown that the upper regions of the brain do not initiate impulses in response to a threatening situation. They are stored as instinctive action and movement patterns, as well as controlled and accessed through the "lower" regions of the brain. Thus, recovering from a trauma and its consequences primarily means being able to master the arousals in the body. Consequently, therapists must become experts in modulating states of arousal. For this purpose, it is absolutely necessary to learn how to deal with our own states of arousal. Only then can we effectively help clients.

HOW DO WE REACH THE SUBCORTICAL BRAIN STRUCTURES?

In order to answer this question, I recommend a look at the animal kingdom. This is precisely what Levine (2010) did, connecting the consequences of a trauma with the immobility reaction. Because this is primarily controlled through the subcortical regions of the brain, animals instinctively end flight or fight reactions that have started, or discharge them through trembling. In this way, they dissipate the compressed energy. For example:

1. A polar bear that is chased by a helicopter and immobilized by an anesthetic shot shows the same reactions as just before the anesthetic shot when it wakes up. Even while it still lies on its back, its paws carry out the running movements. It tries to bite whatever is around it and instinctively completes its fight–flight reaction.

2. If an antelope in the wild is stopped from shaking off this energy after a successful flight, it will not be capable of survival for very long.

The pent-up energy in animals is discharged by ending the defensive strategies with a trembling that can run through the entire body. This prevents traumatization, which would mean immediate death in the world of nature.

This situation is different in human beings. If fight or flight do not succeed, or seem hopeless, the affected person freezes in the defense movement that they can no longer complete—or they dissociate. The energy that has been released for the fight or flight is compressed and tied up in the nervous system. The failed fight and/or unsuccessful flight transforms into helplessness. One reason for this is seen in dissociation.

According to Levine, post-traumatic symptoms are maintained because the defense reaction in the form of intentional movement patterns could not be finished. In physiological terms, every renewed case of freezing is identical with the first experience, but the amount of energy for mastering the situation gets bigger with each additional state of immobility. The immobility reaction not only becomes chronic, but also more intensive. The body is increasingly desperate as it tries to get control over the mobilized energy, but it becomes more and more difficult to end the freezing and dissociation. However, the experiences of energy discharge—no matter whether in the form of trembling, shaking, vibrating, heat, cold, etc.—can be so frightening that the affected person once again dissociates due to the overwhelming feelings (see Levine 2010; Ogden, Minton, and Pain 2006; Rothschild 2002).

These physical states of arousal cannot be ended in a dialog or through logical arguments. If the therapist succeeds in supporting clients in ending the started courses of action that have been frozen in their movement, this will be "understood" by the subcortical brain structures. Immobility (fright) results in a feeling of helplessness, but moving, resisting, or getting to safety triggers feelings of empowerment. So therapists must find a form of communication that makes it possible to reach the body. If clients have the bodily experience of no longer freezing but being able to defend themselves or flee, they get a feeling of empowerment and security. Therapists should be "equipped" for all regions of the brain: the amygdala-controlled emotional and physical movement and action patterns (sensomotoric system), as well as cognitive thought patterns and memory processes. With his Polyvagal Theory, Stephen Porges (2011) provides us with valuable information about how we can "bring" the subcortical brain regions into the therapy and effectively support clients in regulating their states of arousal.

What is sensomotorics? This term is used for the interaction of sensory and motoric capacities, i.e. the management and control of movements in living beings in the interaction with sensory feedback. The perceptions of stimuli through the sensory organs and motor behavior have a direct correlation. Both of these processes run parallel to each other. For example, this would be perception through the eyes and ears and the simultaneously targeted control of arm and foot movements.

POLYVAGAL THEORY

What makes it possible for people to differentiate between safe and threatening situations? How can they know whether a relationship is reliable or not? It is our experiences in the community with others and with certain circumstances that shape our inner maps. These help us to differentiate safe from unsafe relationships and situations, as well as to recognize threatening circumstances. Our nervous system plays an important role in this differentiation. It allows us to engage in three types of behavior: relaxed or stimulating contact, mobilizing the fight-or-flight reaction when in danger, and shutting down as the last way out.

In his *Polyvagal Theory*, Stephen Porges (2011) postulates that our nervous system operates not two but three circuits. On the one hand, we have the sympathetic nervous system and a parasympathetic cord—the nervus vagus. In turn, the latter is divided into a dorsal and ventral branch.

The ventral vagus promotes quiet types of behavior by actively inhibiting the influence of the sympathetic nervous system on the heart. It controls the vocal expression and the ability to listen, but also facial expressions. It enables us to see whether the person in front of us is tense or relaxed. We instinctively register this mood. This means that a relaxed expression and calm voice modulation are basic requirements for us to feel relaxed when we are close to another person.

This immobilization system originates in the brain stem and is called the dorsal motor nucleus of the vagus. We have this cycle in common with almost all of the vertebrates. Due to its continuous conduction, this vagus branch is distinctly slower than the ventral vagus. It starts slowly and switches off just as slowly again. In practice, this means that when we are frozen or dissociated, we need time to "come back" again.

According to Polyvagal Theory, the activation of this cycle to regulate autonomic states follows a hierarchy. We initially try to resolve a situation with our contact system (ventral vagus) by calming the other person through gestures, sounds, or verbal statements. If this does not succeed, the sympathetic nervous system, with its fight-or-flight reaction, is activated. If neither of these leads to success, the oldest system (dorsal vagus) is employed—we give up any type of resistance.

Even before we "know" it, we feel when something is not right. Our brain-stem structures continually monitor the state of our viscera and the performance of our organs such as the heart, lungs, and bowels. As a result, they also support our social behavior.

In order for it to "know" what should be done, our nervous system depends on information from both external and internal sources. Approximately 80 percent of the sensory nerve fibers in our body are occupied with continually keeping our brain supplied with information regarding how we are feeling "in there" in relation to the world "out there." If there is a threat of danger, a motor response will be supported due to the large number of efferent fibers in the direction of the musculature.

Porges postulates that the nervous system receives sensory feedback from receptors that recognize the conditions in the body (interoceptors) and serve to support homeostasis, as well as from receptors that recognize conditions outside of the body (exteroceptors) and serve to master external strains (cf. Porges 2011).

This becomes a problem when an arousal rages in the body, despite nothing happening "out there." Even when the surroundings are safe, the sensory fibers continuously report that there is danger. These stimuli are sent on to the musculature, which reacts to the danger with tension. Through the feedback loop, the motoric fibers report the activity back to the muscles. This creates a never-ending cycle of tension. Or the arousal is so intense that the dorsal vagus "turns on" so that the body becomes flaccid. The person dissociates and gives up.

This understanding of Polyvagal Theory allows us to recognize that the sympathetic nervous system is not activated during every arousal. Due to the fast ventral vagus system, we can be involved and lively at one moment and calm down again at the next. While we start up and shift down, the "vagal brake" inhibits the defense reactions. The social relationship system inhibits both the rise of the sympathetic nervous system and the dorsal vagal complex. This helps us to regulate arising states of arousal in our normal everyday life.

In critical situations, the hierarchy of survival reactions determines our behavior. It allows us to initially look for a solution with relationship-promoting ventrovagal behavior. This includes speaking and placating, but also gestures, postures, and holding eye contact or turning the gaze away. If negotiating and placating do not appear to work, this system resorts to the sympathetic defensive strategies of fight or flight. The body is in uproar, all of the reserves are mobilized, and physical and facial expressions change. Anger or fear is shown in the face, the musculature becomes tense, and the breath becomes flat or is held. If this escape route is also thwarted, there is still the parasympathetic dorsal vagal freeze reaction.

Even if a lot is happening at once, our body is normally good at evaluating whether danger is threatening or not. It knows when it needs to "switch over." Porges calls this process "neuroception."

In people with PTSDs, neuroception is disturbed. They frequently feel endangered in harmless situations. Their defensive strategies are not adequately inhibited or, in other words, the vagal "brake" doesn't function. It may just as well be that they cannot activate their defensive strategies and are therefore not able to bring themselves to safety when they are actually in a threatening situation. Relationship-traumatized children in particular must learn to inhibit their body's sensory feedback in order to be with a threatening caregiver. When those who should offer a sense of emotional security create insecurity, the system of social orientation is disturbed, and the ventrovagal system switches off completely. The vagal brake stops working and the dorsal vagal complex, as well as the sympathetic nervous system, remains alert.

According to Porges, the organism must be made capable of retracting the habitual sympathetic and dorsal vagal reactions. In order for this to occur, the ventrovagal part of the parasympathetic nervous system must be activated to inhibit the sympathetic nervous system and/or the dorsal vagus.

CONSEQUENCES FOR THERAPY

Therapists must consider this factor in therapy if they are to work with people who suffer from complex trauma. The basic prerequisite is that we are capable of inhibiting our own sympathetic nervous system and creating a quiet, open, and relationship-supportive climate. This makes it easier for clients to be in our presence. In order for clients to learn to regulate their affects, it is also indispensable to support them in the development of a healthy neuroception. However, this goal cannot be achieved on a verbal level since the affected regions of the brain cannot be influenced through cognitive or verbal interventions but through sensomotor ones. We communicate with the subcortical brain structures by gently making it possible for clients to feel their body and physical reactions so that they can learn to deal with them but not feel overwhelmed. Clients who cannot perceive their body and/ or avoid being present in their body are not able to benefit from the vagal brake. They remain constantly stuck in the fight-or-flight mode. It is just as essential for the habitually dissociated client to feel their body once again. Only then can they recognize the signs of freezing and dissociation and interrupt the process. The question is, how can the vagal brake be "repaired" or "installed" in clients in the first place?

TOP DOWN VERSUS BOTTOM UP

The choice of the means for overcoming high arousal and coping with a traumatic experience reveals both individual and cultural differences. If we want to make a broad classification, we could say that people imprinted by Western culture tend to explain the reasons for their affects in conversation, and struggle to understand and comprehend them. So the top-down approach is intended to placate their understanding of emotions and body sensations that has been newly acquired in this way. Another path of influence is from the outside to the inside: escaping from the turmoil with drugs, alcohol, prescription drugs, or other distractions.

Far Eastern and African cultures have been familiar with other ways of normalizing arousal for thousands of years. In these cultures people try to regulate their brain from the bottom up since they assume that thoughts and feelings can be influenced by changes in physical sensations. The African strategy consists of dancing and rhythm, and the East relies on tai chi, meditation, qi gong, or yoga. Both cultural spheres use the body.

People process information with a cognitive approach, which is called "top down." When they do this in a sensomotoric and emotional way, this is called "bottom up." But what exactly does this mean?

An example of a top-down approach would be the attentive observation of a situation in which respective individuals focus their attention on areas that are highly likely to contain relevant information (Huestegge 2014). Cognitive processing means that they have developed the ability to observe and assess what they consciously experience, weigh various possibilities, plan, pursue goals, and evaluate results.

We speak of bottom up when the mental processes are exclusively determined by physical stimulus characteristics and not through cognitive integration processes that are language-linked and dependent on learning experiences (Goldstein 2007). Emotional and sensomotoric processing means that individuals experience their emotions and sensations consciously. They observe them and can therefore decide *how* they want to use this information.

Under normal conditions, people are very capable of suppressing feelings such as annoyance or irritation, pain, or hunger, even when their bodies respond with clear signs such as palpitations, muscle contractions, or salivation. They can deliberately ignore these signs and focus on other stimuli. So we can conclude that the "higher" regions of the brain are capable of interrupting or overriding the "lower" ones.

Adults in the West primarily resort to the top-down system. This allows them to perform even under pressure and to make decisions or plans in extreme situations. This type of overriding functions as long as the "upper" regions of the brain control and inhibit the "lower" ones. When this no longer succeeds, the affects can no longer be suppressed or switched off.

When people are plagued by worries or pain that they can no longer suppress or ignore, even with the best will in the world, they experience the same sense of being overwhelmed by their feelings as trauma clients—but in a moderated form. In both cases, the top-down regulation is no longer capable of controlling this occurrence.

SOMATIC MARKERS

But we should not assume that top-down decisions are solely based on reason since every thought and assessment of a situation is linked with a physical sensation. Cognitions cannot be separated from physical experiencing. Somatic markers (Damasio 2006) influence cognitive processing, which helps human beings to structure and simplify the world. Feelings tell people whether or not they should accept a job, for example, and are present when it is necessary to evaluate situations or other people. Depending on how the body reacts to outer stimuli, the physical perception also changes. It accompanies both what is new and what is remembered, marking it as welcome or disruptive. This ability to link body perceptions with stimuli is partly innate and partly developed.

According to Damasio, somatic markers are the basis of these decisions. They make preliminary decisions without individuals being conscious of them. They push human beings in a certain direction or warn them against people and events with which they have already had bad experiences (Lenzen 1997). So somatic markers influence people's decisions and reasoning. Although they believe that they are logically weighing up the possibilities, their background body sensations steer their self-experience and decision-making processes. Beliefs that develop from experience shape people. They are reflected in the body and vice versa.

WHAT CAUSES DISORDERS?

What came first, the chicken or the egg? Applied to our topic, the question is: Do beliefs shape the body or does the latter perpetuate our beliefs? It is certain that physical patterns contribute to the perpetuation of cognitive beliefs and vice versa.

If we consider the development of disorders from a cognitive perspective, overgeneralizations can be the cause for psychological disorders such as depression. Depression is a syndrome that is composed of many individual symptoms. It is expressed verbally, but also in body posture, facial expressions, gestures, voice pitch, and movement patterns. And how does depression develop? The assumption is that there are a series of triggers that are psychologically processed. In turn, this results in the behavior and emotional state of the affected person. But couldn't it happen just as well the other way around, that there was a body posture, gesture, or facial expression in a certain situation that led to a corresponding psychological processing (Niedenthal *et al.* 2009)?

Ogden *et al.* wrote the following:

> If the body shapes reason and beliefs—and vice versa—then the capacity for insight and self-reflection—our ability to "know our own minds"—will be correspondingly limited. How, then, can we begin to know our own minds? If the patterns of the body's movements and posture influence reason, cognitive self-reflection might not be the only or even the best way of bringing the workings of the mind to consciousness. Reflecting on, exploring, and changing the posture and movement of the body may be as valuable. (2006, p.47)

TOP DOWN AND/OR BOTTOM UP?

This allows us to conclude that beliefs can be addressed from two directions: *top down* through cognitive and rational considerations, and *bottom up* through changing the movement and posture patterns.

Top-down therapy concepts such as Cognitive Processing Therapy (CPT) (Resick and Schnicke 1993; Resick, 2011) assume that changes in the cognitions and emotional state also transform the sense of self and the body sense along with it. Ego strengthening plays an important role in the therapeutic process. Narrative Exposure Therapy (NET) (Schauer, Neuner, and Elbert 2011) focuses on transferring the contents stored in the SAM into the VAM, and storing it there through telling a coherent narration. Based on learning theory, the concept of Prolonged Exposure Therapy (PE) (Foa, Hembree, and Rothbaum 2007; Foa, Keane, and Friedman 2000) strives for habituation through the repeated telling and re-experiencing of the traumatic event. These procedures rely on the possibility of cognitively processing the traumatic experience and making it verbally accessible.

As already mentioned above, the sensory trauma memories are "stuck" in the non-verbal subcortical regions of the brain that have no cognitive function. Imaging procedures have clearly shown that the left frontal cortex and the Broca's area—the speech center—experience a functional weakening when PTSD clients remember a trauma. The areas of the right brain hemisphere and the limbic system, which is associated with functions such as emotions, show an increased activity. This particularly applies to the regions around the amygdala.

This finding coincides with the observations that many clients are no longer capable of thinking and speaking during increasing arousal. They can neither explain to themselves nor others what is happening to them. The activity of the right brain hemisphere keeps the affected person entirely trapped in the experiencing, and takes away the possibility of analyzing the event during an arousal.

Brain research has proved that human emotions have their origin in the conditions that predominate in the body. The chemical profile of the body, the state of the inner organs, and the contraction of muscles in the face, throat, abdomen, and extremities—all of this is reported back to the brain. This is assessed and has an effect on the individual's mental state. Talking is absolutely relevant for those who have been traumatized, because they want to comprehend the causes for what has happened and is still happening to them. They were often too young to recognize and evaluate the correlations, or no one was willing to listen to them and believe their stories. Bearing witness, creating correlations, and experiencing one's own existence as a coherent whole—all of this is absolutely necessary for a holistic integration of the traumatic experience.

Pursuing just a top-down approach in trauma therapy to help clients gain insights is not enough, however. Although this may interrupt the automatic physiological alarm reactions, it cannot eliminate them. The perception of why the body reacts in this way and why clients are not capable of stopping these constant experiences of being overwhelmed is an important element in psychoeducation. It becomes easier for clients to relieve their feelings of guilt and shame, as well as understand why they could not have acted any differently in the traumatizing situation. This is also an important element in winning them over for the therapeutic process. More than the intellect is required to heal the disorganized sensations or action patterns of a traumatization. The emotions, sensations, postures, and actions that were frozen at the time of the traumatic event must also be taken into consideration. Only when these individuals are again capable of experiencing their body and biological functions as efficient can they trust them, and therefore themselves, once more. The reawakening of their self-efficacy frequently has a restructuring character, and can positively influence their thinking. In addition, cognitive theories based on exposure therapy can only be effective when clients have learned to better master their affects and body sensations.

WHICH ROLE DO EMOTIONS PLAY?

Let's take a closer look at the role of emotions and the correlation between emotions, cognitions, and their actions. Emotions embody signals that help people to comprehend certain processes such as signs for danger or evidence for safety. Emotions are the driving force for adequate actions because they direct attention to internal and external stimuli. Since traumatized people are generally cut off from their emotions, they also often cannot let themselves be stimulated into taking action by them. Many have become masters in getting through things and practicing self-denial. A female client formulated these circumstances as follows: "I would never have come up with the idea of changing my job or trying to find other work within the company. When they made me the offer to take on a position with more responsibility, I just thought that they know what's right."

Many clients express a lack of interest or display a low level of activity. They tend to experience emotions as reactions to triggers—overwhelming and uncontrollable—that often mislead them into contradictory and rather ineffective actions. They are often not capable of adequately observing or reflecting on emotions in order to use them for decision-making and appropriate actions. Because they do not have the necessary distance to their feelings, they also cannot perceive how emotions develop due to their state of overpowering stress: start, middle, and end. And because they do not experience the end of an affect, they think that they will stay stuck endlessly in something that is intolerable. Avoidance, the inability to think clearly, and/or the inability to differentiate body sensations from emotions in a state of hyperarousal can contribute to them feeling at the mercy of what they have experienced, so new learning and even new evaluating cannot take place.

If the body reacts to triggers with uncontrollable sensations, the body sensation itself becomes a danger since triggers also continue to exist *in* the body after a trauma. Such inner triggers turn the body into a minefield. These physical triggers can assail people at any time and make the trauma into a repetitively occurring current event. The affected people are aware that they shouldn't feel like this, but time and again they are shaken by sensations and feelings that are not tolerable (cf. Emerson and Hopper 2011).

The activities of people who suffer from the symptoms of a traumatization are controlled by the sensomotoric and emotional systems—as in small children. Modulation of behavior is no longer possible in a state of arousal. The clients feel that they are at the mercy of their physical and sensory reactions, as well as their emotional experiencing. They accuse themselves of weakness, and reproach themselves for not being in charge of the situation. This means that the ability for top-down processing is no longer available and the subcortical activity dominates (cf. Ogden *et al.* 2006, p.46).

In order to process a trauma, it must be possible to describe and express the cognitive, emotional, and sensomotoric processes. This is the only way that people can get distance between themselves and what they have experienced. Observing thoughts and emotions—this is something that they may still be familiar with—but turning toward the information from the inner world—perceiving, describing, and expressing physical processes and reactions—tends to be unfamiliar to them. They lack interoception (Latin *inter* "in the middle of" and *recipere* "absorb").

THE INNER WORLD OF THE BODY—THE SIXTH SENSE

> *Interoception* is the perception of processes from inside the body (the perception of the outer world is called *exteroception*). In interoception, only changes in states and not the absolute level of a physiological state are perceived.

The ability to perceive one's own physical sensations was already found to be so relevant by Charles Bell and William James in 1880 that they described it, calling it the "sixth sense" (see Ogden and Minton 2000; Ogden *et al.* 2006). Using the sixth sense means directing the perception inward and comprehending the inner world while the other five senses register the outer world. Through interoceptors, human beings receive information about their location in space (proprioceptors), equilibrium (vestibular system), visceral sensations such as hunger, thirst, palpitations, or nausea (visceroceptors or enteroceptors), pain (nociceptors), or temperature sensations (thermoceptors). In addition, there is a "sense of movement" called the sensation of movement, or kinesthesia.[2]

The "perception of movement," which is perception in relation to one's own movement, can be called a sensory occurrence. The special characteristic of the movement is that it is not controlled by the lower areas of the brain, but by the frontal lobes of the cortex and the motoric and premotor cortex. The brain areas that produce rational thinking and convey the solution for problems also play a role in movements. In 1925, Pierre Janet had already recognized that movements shape the brain and mind—and vice versa (Ogden *et al.* 2006). Science differentiates between movements in a spectrum of unconscious and conscious movements that range from deliberate to involuntary.

TENDENCIES IN MOVEMENTS AND ACTIONS

Human beings learn movements by receiving feedback from the surrounding world. If a sequence of movements does not lead to the desired outcome, it can be changed and adapted until its execution succeeds. This is how we learn to crawl, walk, climb, etc., and continually differentiate our abilities. We develop a movement memory that helps us to automate motoric routines such as brushing our teeth or riding a bicycle. Routines are also created in the interpersonal area. For example, if a family member raises their voice, another person may have a better chance of success by lowering their glance or cowering than by attracting attention. Movement patterns that have an influence on the body structure and the body's functioning develop over time. In turn, these repetitive movement patterns and postures contribute to perpetuating certain thoughts and feelings. If people once again start to perceive themselves and their movements—as well as their own inertia—as their very own actions, they also assume an observer status in relation to the posture and movement. This means that they are capable of having an active influence. The tendencies for action and movement patterns can be changed and integrated as a result. At the same time, new movement patterns represent a different type of self-perception that is a newly structured way of being in the world.

---

2   Kinesthesia means sensation of movements, and is the ability to unconsciously control and direct movements of body parts.

Every *asana* (posture) specifies a structure that can be followed. It initiates a sequence of movements and leads to a certain position that stretches one muscle but activates and strengthens another. For example, when we give instructions on how to do a backbend—which means inviting a client to raise their head, pull their shoulders back, and open their chest—this structured approach involves the opportunity to try out a new posture without addressing a sunken chest or lowered head and "correcting it." We simply practice a posture together, as well as this is possible at the current moment. If the backbend becomes a resource because it feels good to the client, both the *asana* as a sequence of movements and positions, as well as the term "backbend," become an anchor, so to speak. "I can do a backbend at any time when I notice that the pressure on my chest is too much because I'm totally slouching as I sit," a female client commented. "Even if you just say the word 'backbend,' it reminds me that it is possible for me to stretch my muscles and sit up straight. And this immediately feels much better."

In addition, our clients should decide how far they can and want to open up in a backbend. This allows them to cautiously get closer to their feelings and sensations since they decide how they would like to approach this unaccustomed and possibly frightening movement pattern.

INCOMPLETE MOVEMENT PATTERNS

In danger situations, movements are "short-circuited." This means that they are generated by the brain stem. This process enables a lightning-fast automatic reaction and recalling of fixed action patterns. These fixed programs provide relief because they allow a complex sequence of movements to be carried out automatically. An example of this is how drivers step on the brakes and swerve if they see a child running onto the roadway.

However, if the chain of actions is interrupted and the adaptive defensive reaction is stopped, these uncompleted actions can lead to chronic symptoms. In the above example, this could mean that the driver wants to violently jerk the steering wheel to avoid the danger and a collision occurs during this movement. As a result, the defensive strategy was not finished. The movement was not completed and becomes frozen. The fragmentation of the defensive strategy can manifest as constantly tensed musculature in the shoulder and arm or feelings of numbness in the respective body region.

Unfinished defensive actions are also shown in inappropriately aggressive, fearful, or passive behavior. A client told me that he could fly off the handle for such trivial reasons that it caused the people around him to tremble and hide at the sight of him. His body reacts to the former danger signals involuntarily, and carries out the movements automatically, "so things sometimes also fly through the room."

Inappropriately fearful behavior can be expressed in that the affected person does not feel safe during the day. A female client reported: "During the lunch break, when I have to leave my office to get something to eat, I need at most ten minutes to do this. I often don't realize what I bought until I'm back in the office."

The question as to why an adult woman would behave like this in the middle of the day is answered by the following episode from her childhood: "My route to school was like a horror trip. Other students would lie in wait and beat me up. They took my school things and hid or destroyed them. Walking out of the classroom or home always meant leaving a secure place that offered me a minimum of safety." In order to protect herself, she had developed the habit of quickly making a beeline for her destination, and attracting as little attention as possible on the way.

In both of these cases, movements were carried out for no reason, and a dissociative state predominated. The action patterns run automatically. It is not possible for the person to analyze the situation at that moment—the bottom-up regulation inhibits the cognitive top-down processing.

These action tendencies are stored in the procedural memory (SAM) and displayed in conditioned behavior (Ogden *et al.* 2006). Such conditioned action sequences do not require images, motivations, or cognitive representations to be carried out. The automated action tendencies become part of the personal behavior, even if the external conditions long belong to the past.

For trauma treatment, this means promoting the awareness of body sensations, observing action tendencies, and supporting clients in being able to perceive themselves (Levine 2010; Ogden and Minton 2000; Rothschild 2002). If clients are capable of feeling their body, as well as observing and describing their physical reactions, this increases the chances that they will no longer experience their behavior as remote-controlled or directed by others, but can control and integrate it on their own. The focus of the therapy shifts to the body since cognitive and emotional experiences do not occur without a physical correspondence.

WHAT DOES BRAIN RESEARCH SAY?

When considering interoception from the perspective of neuroscience, and asking once again about access to the brain stem and limbic structures, this yields the following answers: The dorsolateral prefrontal cortex houses the working memory. This is where plans for actions are prepared, yet there are no connections with the emotional brain. Although people can critically grapple with lacking a sense of wellbeing, analyzing this does not affect any kind of change in the primary feelings (fear and panic, anger and rage, or disgust). However, the medial prefrontal cortex is active in the experience of self-awareness and sensing of the self. This part of the brain is coupled with the amygdala and has access to the emotional brain. So if self-awareness is activated through interoception, it is possible to access emotions and therefore the subcortical brain structures.

4

WHAT TO DO?

STABILIZATION OR EXPOSURE THERAPY?

Trauma exposure is an important element in the therapy, which has been proven by numerous studies. However, not every client can handle the stress of remembering. This is why any adequately long period of stabilization is recommended at the start of the therapy for people with complex trauma. This is followed by the exposure phase, working through the traumatic occurrence, and its integration. These stages are not independent units—the process often consists of jumping forward and back between the various phases.

But there are also other opinions. Petzold (1996) points out that the research on the practice of trauma exposure shows anything but clear results. According to Petzold, bringing a client's suppressed trauma into consciousness at any price includes the danger of a harmful obsession when ignoring the fact that avoidance or suppression can represent meaningful and effective coping strategies. Forcing the remembering of a trauma can intensify pathological hyperarousal patterns and lead to negative effects (cf. also van der Kolk 2009). Symptoms such as numbing can be intensified by forcing clients to work through them. Therapists must be capable of careful diagnosis, and offer flexible intervention strategies as well as different treatment techniques in order to let clients feel safe and not in danger (cf. Petzold 1996).

Therapists should therefore have a repertory of intervention possibilities that is as broad as possible so that they can respond to clients and select an appropriate approach. An exposure brings harmful consequences with it when clients have an excessive level of stress without knowing how to calm themselves and find their way back to their personal "window of tolerance." So the baby should not be thrown out with the bathwater by making exposure therapy responsible for harmful consequences.

Instead, the errors should primarily be sought in the insufficient preparation and/or stabilization of clients. Many trauma victims suffer from such a high stress level that a therapy is generally difficult for them. Even just the path to the practice and the confrontation with the therapist is an effort. On the one hand, they are afraid, but on the other, they know that this will involve emotional injuries from their past. And this puts many clients into the highest state of alert. They need all of their resources to keep their sensations and feelings in check. They often already dissociate before the session due to the high arousal so that they are unable to benefit from the therapy. Dissociative moments can partially or completely erase their memory of the session's contents.

According to Bessel van der Kolk:

> If it is true that at the core of our traumatized and neglected clients' disorganization is the problem that they cannot analyze what is going on when they re-experience the physical sensations of past trauma, but that these sensations just produce intense emotions without being able to modulate them, then our therapy needs to consist of helping people to stay in their bodies and to understand these bodily sensations. And that is certainly not something that any of the traditional psychotherapies…help people to do very well. (quoted in Rothschild 2002, p.20)

In order to achieve this stabilization, therapists must explain to clients in a first step, by means of a detailed and repeated psychoeducation, that their bodily reactions are normal processes. In a second step, therapists must support clients in becoming familiar with their bodies in a cautious way. Clients become more secure once they start to understand that their symptoms are not an expression of their weakness or abnormality. In a further step, therapists require techniques that allow clients to improve their affect regulation. When traumatized people literally experience in their own bodies that they can have a direct influence on their wellbeing and calm themselves with a breathing exercise, posture, or physical movement, this initiates an increase of empowerment, confidence, and self-assurance. The arousal symptoms take place in the body. Since these are often split off and/or rejected, it is important to help clients reduce the relationship to their bodies that is characterized by negation, anger, helplessness, or hate. Instead, the focus can shift to care and connectedness with their own corporeality.

For those affected, developing a relationship with their own bodies is just as challenging as creating sustainable and trusting contacts with other people. So should we first be concerned with a stable relationship?

FIRST DEVELOP A GOOD RELATIONSHIP

Since many triggers develop within the scope of interpersonal contacts, it is not easy for clients with complex traumatization to trust in and open up to someone. It is understandable that relationships represent minefields for clients because they predominately feel mistrust and vigilance after bad experiences. The creation of a sustainable therapeutic relationship can only succeed when clients possess a certain degree of affect regulation in order to deal with the triggers that are inevitably provoked in the treatment. Therapists are interested in a constructive and trusting cooperation, but if they only pay attention to building a sustainable therapeutic relationship, they may become part of the client's dysfunctional relationship pattern. Why? Because they try to avoid everything that could destroy security and trust.

So clients require functioning tools that help them to calm themselves. Only then can they deal with the stress that is undeniably triggered by a therapeutic relationship. At the least, they can trust us, as therapists, to the extent that we take them seriously, understand their symptoms, explain the correlations, and give them a functioning strategy that provides tangible relief.

WHICH FORM OF THERAPEUTIC RELATIONSHIP IS ADVISABLE?

Which ideas exist on the topic of shaping a therapeutic relationship? One idea is that a trusting therapeutic relationship is the medicine that helps people to develop and heal. It enables regression and reparenting, allowing clients to have new experiences in the therapy relationship. They can try something out, receive feedback on their behavior, and consequently gain the opportunity to shape their relationships more satisfactorily in the future (Lenzinger-Bohleber, Roth, and Buchheim 2008).

According to a different, Buddhist-oriented concept, human beings have everything that they need to master their own lives. But their access to this ability may be blocked. In keeping with this thought model, the guru or master guides clients in making their personal resources accessible and useful to them. This approach is now found in coaching.

Whether we use one of these two models—or even a completely different one—as the basis of our treatment formula is up to us alone and based on our own mentality. Let's consider the two basic attitudes outlined above from the perspective of treating clients with complex PTSDs. As we know from experience, our relationship offer can awaken memories of previous relationships in the clients. They regress and live out their old relationship patterns in the therapy. However, it is counterproductive—especially at the start of the therapy—to bring people with complex trauma into a regressive state. This is an uncontrollable, dangerous situation for them and will strain the therapeutic relationship at a later point. On the other hand, if we just see ourselves as coaches who stay outside and instruct the clients, this can lead to a difficult (or disturbing) relationship and lack of contact.

However, if we open up a transitional space in which the pathology and post-maturing can be explored (Reddemann 2001), this has a relieving effect for both sides. Many clients can deal with this *space of possibilities* in a better way since this is where they experience "normality" and therefore stability (Sachsse and Roth 2008).

THE THIRD SPACE

If we work with the metaphors of possibility spaces, we can differentiate between three of them. The first space involves the inner emotional processes, which is the relationship with the self. In the second space, a relationship arises that is contact with other people. The third space is one of transition or possibilities in which something different can happen, such as imagination, play, or dance (Reddemann 2001). In this space, there is no right or wrong, no failure, and no defamation. It is a space that allows us to try things out, correct them, and attempt them again. Transitional spaces can be experienced in play therapy, through imagination, in concentrative movement therapy, and in body-oriented forms of therapy such as yoga, qi gong, or Feldenkrais, as well as in art and expressive therapy.

If we take the idea of the space of possibilities seriously in body-oriented trauma therapy, this space must not focus on the "right" postures or movements. I understand "right" here as perfect postures, "acrobatic" *asanas*, and movements that are immediately corrected. It is not an honest play space when something must be achieved, when someone stands over a person and says what should be done, and when someone evaluates whether it was done well. This is a hierarchical relationship and not one on an equal footing. And it is a familiar relationship pattern, to which clients can only react with the habitual strategies: submissive adaptation, cynical resistance, or dissociation.

Klinkenberg (2007) wrote the following in his German-language book on mindfulness in body behavioral therapy:

> All of the methods that are based on "right" or "wrong" actions easily fall short, even if they simultaneously take into consideration the one or the other very justifiable aspect of movement behavior. The sensomotoric structure of human beings does not correspond with doing, a certain action, or a posture that should be assumed. Instead, human possibilities are virtually dependent on demands, suggestions, and experiencing to come into play.

And he postulated:

> It is therefore also important to leave the questions of a clarifying attempt open in such a way that we are free for surprises: Even the thousandth attempt should be approached so impartially that new and still undiscovered things can still interest me... [This should] occur without any intention of following a specific goal—also and especially when we have already experienced how this has had an effect during an earlier attempt. (2007, p.24ff.)

A female client who attended my yoga groups gave me the following feedback:

> As I sat on the pillow and heard that I should try to direct my focus to the movement of the breath, I thought that I would immediately have a panic attack and then pass out. I was certain that I couldn't do this. Then I heard that when my thoughts wander off or I get lost in a daydream, I can simply bring my focus back to the movement or observe my thoughts or daydreams—in whatever way that I would like to do this. "There is no failure," I heard you say, "because as soon as you notice that your thoughts are drifting off, you are already

being mindful because you notice it. And…mindfully observing our thoughts is also mindfulness." I had never heard anything like this. I instantly relaxed and could really observe the movements of my breath—for a while. But I didn't feel bad because I couldn't do this for long. Being given permission like this was something completely new for me.

Yoga opens up a transitional space where creative exploration becomes possible. Practicing and exploring together allows clients to come into or stay in a relationship with themselves in the presence of another person. And this works because we are in a relationship with ourselves and observe our own interoception, which we share with the clients but never assess, evaluate, or prescribe what they should feel. There are no requirements of the relationship. This allows trauma clients to get an impression of what it feels like to be neither alone nor lost, and also not to have to be on guard and to protect themselves.

At this point I would like to once again ask the question of "stabilize or expose?" As trauma therapists, we must honestly engage with the following questions: Do we avoid the exposure together with clients because we ourselves are fearful and uncertain? Is this why we are avoiding it to focus on stabilization and the development of the relationship? Or is the affected client really not yet capable of tolerating the memories?

The transitional space removes these questions. By inviting clients to explore, try things out, and have experiences together with us in terms of what kinds of effects breathing and physical exercises have, we realize both. We expose the habitual split-off body, virtually put it back into the focus of the attention, and use it for stabilization, as well as for the regulation of affects and self-regulation. A subsequent exposure of the trauma memories—which makes cognitive and emotional integration possible in addition to somatic integration—therefore becomes more tolerable for both parties.

PART II

EAST: CONNECTING BODY AND MIND

5

YOGA IS MORE THAN *ASANAS*

Yoga has been gaining momentum in the Western world for years. The experience of hectic everyday life has awakened the need for physical relaxation and inner collection within many people. But most adepts are not aware of the synthesis between physical techniques and spiritual components.

I would like to invite you to expand your knowledge of yoga, because it is more than physical fitness and a workout such as in power yoga or assuming sometimes challenging positions.

HISTORY AND PRINCIPLES

The discipline of yoga, a "path of liberation," developed in India over the millennia within the context of its main religions: Hinduism, Buddhism, and Jainism. The goal of yoga practice is escaping the wheel of karmic reincarnation. The four first sutras of the work by Patanjali (2010) summarize the yoga path in the following way: Yoga is inner silence.

The Sanskrit word *yoga* means the "harnessing" or "yoking" of draft animals to a cart (Fuchs 2007). From the perspective of yoga, a person's five senses and drives must be yoked in order to achieve the state of pure being and pure perception, and therefore attaining enlightenment. The *Bhagavad Gita*, a sacred scripture of the Hindu faith, has the image of a chariot (the body) drawn by five horses (five senses), which the charioteer (the soul) should learn to control (Hawley 2002).

On a practical level, yoga means balancing the body, mind, and emotions. If there is an imbalance on the physical, mental, or emotional level, the natural interaction between muscles, nerves, and organs is lost. The practice of yoga is intended to restore this alignment so that all of the components work together harmoniously. Yoga is neither a religion nor a doctrine but a collection of methods that gives its practitioners instructions in how to achieve this balance once again (Fuchs 2007).

In India, the practice of yoga means the systematic training of the body and mind through inner collection. Redemptive perceptions or redemption itself should be achieved through direct experiencing.

The tradition of yoga can look back on a history of more than 3000 years and has produced an entire series of practice paths. All of these paths follow the same goal: unification with God, enlightenment (*samadhi*), and therefore escape from the wheel of reincarnation.

PATHS TO LIBERATION

There are four main paths in yoga that support reaching this goal:

- *Karma yoga,* the yoga of works. Practitioners refrain from any selfish interests or worldly results in all of their activities. They do not act for the sake of their action's fruits but sacrifice the results to the sublime.

- *Jnana yoga,* the yoga of realization and knowledge. Through the striving for realization and truth, practitioners achieve redemption from the cycle of reincarnation. In modern terms, this is a top-down strategy.

- *Bhakti yoga,* the yoga of devotion to God. The cultivation of an intensive relationship and love of the chosen deity, as well as a devotional practice with an emphatically emotional dedication, is intended to lead practitioners to a lack of desires and to liberation.

- *Raja yoga,* the yoga of mastering the senses. Practitioners strive for a step-by-step development and mastery of the mind. Another term for Raja yoga is Ashtanga yoga, literally, "eight-limbed."

THE EIGHTFOLD PATH OF RAJA YOGA

Raja yoga is the basis of modern yoga practice and serves as the foundation for this book. The customary and familiar yoga practices are found in the Eightfold Path: *asanas* (body postures), *pranayama* (consciously directed breathing), and meditation. In addition, the path of yoga includes further practical instructions such as withdrawal of the senses and collection or concentration. It provides practitioners with rules for their attitude toward life in general and their own existence in particular. Practitioners achieve mastery over the mind through self-observation and self-analysis. They recognize their individual patterns, learn what limits their potential and what is beneficial for them, and how to orient their actions upon this.

ELEMENTS OF THE EIGHTFOLD PATH OF RAJA YOGA (CF. FUCHS 2007)

1. Five *yamas*, the five rules of general order.

2. Five *niyamas* include the five rules of special order.

3. *Asana* was originally the correct sitting posture or "calm" posture.

4. *Pranayama* can be translated as mindful breathing.

5. *Pratyahara* is withdrawing the senses.

6. *Dharana* means collection or concentration.

7. *Dhyana* stands for pure observation or meditation.

8. *Samadhi*, the goal, is oneness or enlightenment.

If we take a close look at the rules, they seem quite contemporary and can serve us as orientation in modern everyday life.

THE FIVE *YAMAS* REGULATE OUR DEALINGS WITH OTHERS

THE FIVE *YAMAS*

- *Satya*—truthfulness: Being truthful means not lying to ourselves and also admitting unpleasant things to ourselves.

- *Ahimsa*—non-violence: Peaceful behavior is not the same as not being allowed to defend ourselves. Instead, this concerns cultivating a well-considered way of interacting with all living beings and with ourselves.

- *Asteya*—non-stealing: We should not take what doesn't belong to us, either in the material or the spiritual sense.

- *Aparigraha*—non-avarice: This means only taking what is appropriate. It also includes not exploiting any presumably "favorable" opportunities.

- *Brahmacharya*—not allowing ourselves to be distracted from the path: As yogis, we should organize our life and relationships to people and things so that they promote our striving for wisdom.

Ahimsa (non-violence), the second rule, which is also stressed by Emerson and Hopper (2011), requires a more extensive explanation, since it represents a main aspect of TSY. *Ahimsa* means friendliness in thoughts, words, and actions. This means that we should not force anyone, not even ourselves, to do something that we do not want to do or that is not beneficial for us. The "sporty" side of yoga hardly considers *ahimsa*. Whenever people are pushed or pulled in the "right" direction or spurred on to more perseverance, this is no longer about a cautious and curious exploring of boundaries. If we constantly overstep them, this is actually a form of violence. Being a role model is the best way to communicate the friendly attitude to our students and clients.

Here is an example from practice that illustrates the effect of *ahimsa.* After an hour of TSY, I received the following feedback: "Today I only did as much as I could without feeling any pain and any exaggerated exertion. This was entirely differently for me—completely new! I believe that I don't even know my boundaries and only encounter them when I feel pain."

Ahimsa leads us to an inner attitude that also has an effect on the relationship with our clients. By leaving the control over how to perform the exercises up to them at all times, they can have new experiences in contrast to their previous understanding of bonding.

THE FIVE *NIYAMAS* RELATE TO HOW WE TREAT OURSELVES

THE FIVE *NIYAMAS*

- *Sauca*—purity/hygiene, in both the physical and spiritual sense: This means maintaining healthy body functions, as well as achieving spiritual clarity. *Asana* and *pranayama* are considered essential means for achieving inner purity.

- *Santosha*—contentment, modesty, and satisfaction: This means taking things as they are.

- *Tapas*—heating: Disciplined and sustained practice of the *asanas* and *pranayama* "heat" the body, which can rid itself of "waste" in this way by stoking the inner fire (*agni*).

- *Svadhyaya*—study of the self: Observing our own thinking and actions and critically questioning them in order to become more conscious.

- *Ishwarapranidhana*—trust in God: It is enough to know that we have done our best, then we can confidently put the rest into God's hands.

The *niyamas* provide valuable information for life in general and yoga practice in particular. *Santosha* (contentment) is explained in greater detail here. Since people in the West have entirely different moral concepts, we are very much in danger of developing false ambitions for both ourselves and our clients. *Santosha* encourages us not to compare ourselves with others and to have no expectations of the results. If we do yoga with ambition and a results orientation, we will certainly encounter familiar patterns. We make comparisons and torment ourselves with accusations if we "do worse" than others. In TSY, we explore our perceptions in the *asanas*. Instead of striving for a certain goal, we experience every moment as it is. If we practice in this way, there are no errors since what we observe is neither right nor wrong—it is an experience.

ASANA

Asana originally meant the quiet sitting posture in which yogis meditate. Once the body was seen as a means of liberation, further positions developed to make a higher level of mindfulness possible and to facilitate a stable basis for exploring the breath, the body, the mind, and being.

PRANAYAMA

The ancient yogis observed that they could have a direct influence on their nervous system through breath control or breath mindfulness— and therefore on their mental states. Based on this insight, they developed both stimulating and calming *pranayama* exercises.

Asana and *pranayama*, the third and fourth steps of the Eightfold Path, will be discussed in more detail later (see Chapters 13 and 14) since both play a main role in TSY.

PRATYAHARA

With the fifth step of *pratyahara*, we cross the middle of the Eightfold Path. This signifies the transition from the outer to the inner aspects of yoga and is associated with the "mastering of outside influences." In our commercially oriented world, our senses are constantly bombarded by stimuli that distract and lead people to consumption. If we do not get them under control, they plague us with endless demands. Like a turtle that avoids the dangers of its surrounding world by retracting its head, we can decide to repel the external stimuli for a certain time. This conscious act should not be equated with avoiding triggers, which is something that trauma clients have generally mastered in an exceptional way. The mastering of outside influences is a deliberate process. We train the ability to control our senses when we practice *asanas* or *pranayama* by bringing our attention back to a certain focus time and again after every distraction. So we learn to be increasingly better at dealing with stimuli.

DHARANA

Dharana means concentration. We narrow our focus and direct our attention to something like a point in the body, the movement of the breath, a mantra, the void, or God. Every step of the yoga path sets the course for the next. So we already prepare for *dharana* through the practice of *pratyahara* on a regular basis. *Pratyahara* relieves and liberates from the stimuli that assault us from the outside so that we can direct our attention entirely at one single point. The longer concentration (*dharana*) leads to meditation (*dhyana*).

DHYANA

The term *dhyana* emphasizes undisturbed concentration, meditation, and pure, mindful observation. If the state of *dharana* stands for "targeted" attention focused on an object, "undisturbed" concentration counts on the level of *dhyana*. Instead of having to focus on the breathing, a mantra, or an object, the concentration required in *dhyana* gradually fades. What remains is pure consciousness or clarity. The mind is so still in this state that no more thoughts arise in this peace of mind.

SAMADHI

Samadhi is the state of oneness, which is the final purpose of every yoga path. The striving of TSY is certainly not to achieve enlightenment, yet brief moments of inner silence and oneness can become valuable resources.

For traumatized people, contemplation and meditation can mean that they are at the mercy of all their memories and fears. This means that we, trauma therapists, prefer a form of "meditation in motion" that allows us to concentrate on one physical aspect, so clients can stay in the here and now, which diffuses the pull of their traumatic past. It would be even more correct to speak of "collection or mindfulness in motion."

"Perceiving without reacting" must also be approached in a differentiated manner. It is important to differentiate between what kinds of things people react to. If someone's knee hurts, we should absolutely react and change the position or end the *asana*. Communicating the concept of *dhyana* without reflection to trauma clients can conjure up their old behavior patterns so that they just hold out again and do not react. We encourage our clients to respond to their perceptions and personally decide in which position, for how long, and in which intensity they want to perform an *asana*. When applied to affects, the ability of purely observing emotions and the corresponding physical reactions without needing to respond to them (*dhyana*) *is a goal worth striving for—and not just for trauma clients.*

6

"WORK-IN"— HATHA YOGA

Hatha yoga is the form of yoga that is most familiar in the West. Hatha means "strength," which should highlight the physical and mental exertion that must be applied to achieve this goal. For example, *ha* is translated to mean the Sun and *tha* as the Moon, as the male and female, hot and cold, to symbolize the polarity of all being or opposite energies. The teachings of Hatha yoga see the body as the temple of God, which must be given appropriate attention to keep it healthy. The exercises are intended to strengthen the body, keep it supple, and perfect its natural aptitudes.

On the Eightfold Path, physical exercises are found on steps 3 and 4. The first two steps of Raja yoga—*yamas* and *niyamas*, following the rules of life—represent a hurdle for some adepts and block their path to liberation. However, the mind can transform itself, and the rules of life can easily become self-evident through practicing *asanas* on a regular basis. This opens the path of liberation to everyone.

We can see that the possibility of changing mental processes through practicing postures and breath control is not a new approach. And this is precisely what TSY is about. By practicing body awareness with our clients, we trust that their attitudes and beliefs will change. So yoga is a bottom-up approach, a path from the outside to the inside. In other words, it is a "work-in."

By mindfully practicing on a regular basis, not only the occurrences of the body and breath are changed but the continued concentration also trains the consciousness. By becoming aware of their restless mind, practitioners recognize that this state scatters their energy and that they rarely stay in their center. Through this practicing, they experience moments of inner silence, which awakens the wish to experience this type of collection more frequently (cf. Fuchs 2007). Anyone who has already tried to meditate knows how difficult it is to keep the mind quiet since it constantly gets lost in daydreams, worries, and plans. The pure awareness, this lingering in the here and now, sounds so simple, yet at the beginning, we only achieve it for seconds or at best for a few minutes after some practice time. Time and again, we lose control of ourselves.

7

THE TOOLS OF A YOGI

ASANA

The original meaning of *asana* was "seat" or "sitting posture." The ancient sources say that the seat should be firm and pleasant. This sitting posture serves the complete relaxation and contemplation of the infinite. It is conspicuous that assuming this *asana* did not originally serve to help people experience their body more intensively, make it more flexible, or develop a better physical consciousness. The sitting posture was the means to redemption. It meant an ascetic posture, the Bound Lotus—people sit in the Lotus Seat with their arms crossed behind their back and hold the forward sections of their feet. In this position, it was considered important to stay absolutely calm. Such a standstill can be understood as imitating the mode of being for the pure mind and complete concentration on oneself (cf. Fuchs 2007).

New aspects were only added later with the understanding of the body as the temple of the divine. In Hatha yoga, the *asanas* were used as a contribution to higher mindfulness and a stable basis for enabling exploration of the breath, the body, the mind, and being.

Many *asanas* have animal names like the Cobra, Cat, Cow, Hare, etc. People who lived in and with nature observed how the animals had an existence in harmony with their surroundings and their body. They tried to put themselves into the positions of certain animals in order to discover that these postures created a change in their being and experiencing. For example, when they imitated a hare, they felt the flow of adrenaline responsible for the fight or flight reflex, and recognized that they could influence it—which is an astonishing parallel to the goals of trauma therapy. This imitation of animal postures helped them to encounter the challenges of nature (cf. Swami Satyananda Saraswati 2010, p.10).

Further *asanas* developed that reflected the conflicts with interpersonal manifestations such as the Warrior or Hero and those of nature such as the Tree and the Rock. The goal has always been to explore the nature of the mind in order to ultimately achieve *samadhi*— enlightenment.

Modern yoga has developed endless varieties so that we can now find the appropriate *asanas* for us, and vary them until they correspond with our personal mental state.

The yogic work is different from sports training not only through the mental attitude of the practitioners, who carry out the movements with mindfulness and concentration; *asanas* also activate completely different bodily mechanisms than something like gymnastic exercises. During the practice of the *asanas*, the breathing and metabolism slow down, and oxygen consumption and body temperature decrease. The opposite occurs during sports: oxygen consumption and body temperature rise.

The *asanas* can be divided into the following groups:

- standing and sitting postures

- forward bends, side bends, and backbends

- twists

- reverse positions

- balance exercises

- relaxation positions

- static and dynamic *asanas*.

The practice section (see Part V) has photos and instructions for *asanas* in various degrees of difficulty using a chair and in standing positions. It is important not to see the *asanas* as a rigid concept. They offer us countless variations for experiencing the body in creative possibilities of expression, and train a curious and non-judgmental observer status.

PRANAYAMA

Especially for trauma clients, access to breathing—which is always also access to the emotions—succeeds more easily through observation of the breathing movement than a concept of purely "observing the breath."

A female client said that:

> …breath is dangerous… The breath inevitably leads to the emotions. But it is possible to observe the breath movement. Over time, I managed to get better and better at perceiving the breath as such and tolerating the affects that arise with it. If we had started with it in the training, I would not have been able to endure it.

When we consider breath control from the perspective of yoga, we find it on the fourth step of the Eightfold Path.

Pranayama consists of two words, *prana* and *ayama*. *Prana* can best be translated as "energy." *Ayama* means something like lengthening, expansion, control, and non-dissipation, as well as the free flowing that is no longer controlled by the will. So *pranayama* also indicates the expansion, regulation, and free flowing of *prana* or energy. Although the ancient yogis did not have modern anatomical and physiological knowledge or our examination possibilities available to them, their attention was focused on the occupation with breathing. According to their understanding, the breath represents the connection between body and mind. *Pranayama*—breathing exercises that control the mind and support presence in the here and now—is an essential component of yoga.

Practitioners achieve control over the mind through self-observation and self-analysis. They recognize their individual patterns and discover what limits or benefits their potential. This is what they orient their actions upon.

If we consider the various forms of *pranayama*, the exercises can be classified into the following:

- stimulating or sympathetic

- calming or parasympathetic

- balancing exercises, or those that create balance between the sympathetic and parasympathetic nervous system

- dynamic breathing exercises that are performed in combination with a movement

- breathing exercises that are connected with a tone or sound.

The practice section (see Part V) contains concrete instructions and examples of how to include breath and the related awareness of the breath into the therapeutic practice. The inner attitude with which we perform both the *asanas* and *pranayama* can best be described as mindfulness.

MINDFULNESS

The dictionary lists the following synonyms for the word "mindfulness": attention, focus, preciseness, thoroughness, interest, concentration, collection, care, participation, circumspection, caution, and vigilance. My impression is that it is difficult for Western thinking to understand the meaning of this word.

Seen in historical terms, mindfulness (called *sati* in the Pali language) can primarily be found in the Buddhist teachings and meditation practice (Vipassana meditation), and represents the basis of the attention-based attitude in the meditative practices of all Buddhist traditions. The term *sati* is translated as mindfulness or presence of mind. But everyday language does not have a term that completely corresponds with the significance of *sati* because the Buddhist understanding of it ranges far beyond the ordinary understanding of attention or presence of mind. A definition by Kabat-Zinn is frequently used for mindfulness. He says that mindfulness "means paying attention in a particular way; on purpose, in the present moment, and nonjudgmentally" (2007, p.75). Mindfulness solely has the goal of acknowledging the contents of current consciousness. It does not strive for a specific state such as relaxation or a change in arising feelings (Bishop *et al.* 2004).

The Eightfold Path describes the withdrawal of the senses— *pratyahara*—and learning collection and/or concentration—*dharana*— as aids or preliminary stages for pure observation and meditation. Withdrawal of the senses means that we take our attention away from the surrounding world. If we see, hear, or perceive something through other sensory channels, we do not allow it to have any attention and significance but remain in or return to the awareness of the breath, the body, or whatever we are focusing on at the moment. For people who suffer from hypervigilance, this is initially an unsolvable task and challenge that seems insurmountable. But they can approach it step by step within a safe framework. Concentration, or, in the language of the Eightfold Path, collection, is not only indispensable in doing this exercise, but it also serves as an aid.

TECHNIQUES FOR CULTIVATING MINDFULNESS

All meditative traditions teach the judgment-free contemplation of the constantly changing internal and/or external stimuli. They show adepts the transience of the stimuli, as well as the reactions (Hart 1987; Kabat-Zinn 1990). If the attention drifts away, it is brought back to the respective object of attention as soon as the practitioner becomes aware of this.

The forms vary from meditating in the sitting position (Hart 1987) to alternating between a sitting and walking meditation (Kabat-Zinn 1990; Mahasi Sayadaw 1971). The focus of attention also differs. The thoughts and sensations can be labeled (Mahasi Sayadaw 1971), and the sensations can be observed in the tradition of body sweeping. Or the breath and sensation of the breath can be used as objects of attention (Hart 1987).

If we consider mindfulness under the aspects of yoga, we find many possibilities for developing the mindful observation of interoceptive processes. For example, these can be seen in:

- movements of the breath

- movement of the body

- muscle activity such as tension, stretching, etc.

- changes in the musculature, breath, etc. after an *asana*

- the perception of the body in space: "Where is my arm? Where are my knees?" and so forth

- kinesthetic sensations such as the structure of the floor, etc.

- temperature differences

- the weight of one body part or the body itself.

This intentional attention in non-judgmental openness may lead to a change of perspective. The better practitioners become at letting go of the contents of consciousness and just observing them, the less they will be "swept away" by them. We experience the contents of consciousness as something that is constantly changing and transient. In a certain sense, this creates a gap—a space between the sensations and reactions to them (Hölzel 2007). Practitioners train themselves to deal with the situation in a reflected way instead of reacting reflexively (Bishop *et al.* 2004). All of these are desirable goals for individuals who are overwhelmed by frequent, uncontrollable affects.

PART III

WEST STUDIES EAST: RESEARCH

8

YOGA HELPS!

There must be something to it when millions of people in the world now practice yoga, and more than 150 studies conducted in the USA and India (although not all can be seen as strictly empirical) provide evidence on the usefulness of yoga in a great variety of health issues. There are studies on how yoga has a positive influence on individual states of mind, cardiovascular disorders such as hypertension, the respiratory system, sympathetic overexcitation, concentration, and a subjective sense of wellbeing (Khalsa Dharma Singh and Stauth 2004). With regard to moods and emotional wellbeing, scientists presume that *pranayama* and other mindfulness techniques make it easier for practitioners to identify their negative thoughts and to distance themselves from them so that they can examine them for their validity (Segal, Williams, and Teasdale 2002). The emotions that accompany the thoughts can shift into something positive this way. Some authors presume that the ability for self-soothing creates a positive effect (Kissen and Kissen-Kohn 2009; Waelde, Thompson, and Gallagher-Thompson 2004).

Other body-oriented approaches that can be integrated into psychotherapy show promising results. Examples of these are progressive muscle relaxation (Delgado *et al.* 2010), deep breathing (Arch and Craske 2006), rhythm and dance (Berrol 1992), or meditation (Salmon *et al.* 2004). Yoga unites many of these above-mentioned interventions: breathing, mindfulness, meditation, and rhythmic movement.

YOGA INFLUENCES NEUROTRANSMITTERS

A much-quoted fascinating study on the effect of yoga was conducted by scientist Chris Streeter and her team (Streeter *et al.* 2007). They measured the GABA (gamma-aminobutyric acid) level in subjects—all of who practiced different yoga styles—before and after a one-hour yoga session. In the meantime, a control group occupied itself with magazines and light fiction. The result showed that the GABA level of the yoga group rose by an average of 27 percent. In the most experienced yogis and yoginis, or those who practiced intensively, a downright wave of GABA had started (Streeter *et al.* 2007). Streeter and her team then wanted more precise information: Was it yoga or the physical activity that brought about these results? In a further study they compared yoga with walking, and found that GABA rose in both groups, although the GABA values were higher in the beginner yogis and yoginis than in the walking group (Streeter *et al.* 2010).

GABA (GAMMA-AMINOBUTYRIC ACID)

GABA is the most important inhibiting neurotransmitter in the brain. In quiet, stress-free phases, it inhibits the glutamate transmission (glutamate is an amino acid, and the most important stimulating neurotransmitter in the brain) to regions of the brain such as the thalamus and amygdala. It helps the brain to filter out irrelevant information. However, an elevated glutamate level can lead to the elimination of GABA inhibition in phases of stress, and trigger a cascade of protective reactions.

GABA has a relaxing and anxiety-relieving effect. A stress-induced rise in glutamate enables cortical and subcortical communication. The latter is necessary in order to react to danger. However, an elevated glutamate level can result in extreme changes in the intracellular system to the point of cell death. In order to protect the brain, GABA is therefore also released in stress situations.

The plasma level of GABA is an indicator for depression and PTSD. A number of studies detected lower GABA levels in individuals who had developed PTSD after a disaster than in test people who did not exhibit any PTSD after the event. It has not yet been possible to prove whether GABA is a protective factor, or whether people with higher GABA values have a lowered vulnerability (Vaiva *et al.* 2004).

There is no doubt that trauma clients would benefit from higher GABA levels. Vaiva and his team (2004) hypothesized that lower GABA levels increase susceptibility for PTSD after an exposure to trauma. The team studied 108 victims of traffic accidents, and discovered that the GABA levels of victims with PTSD symptoms were significantly lower than those without. Provided that the GABA level is genetically determined, this study leads to the conclusion that people with a lower GABA level have a higher risk of developing PTSD under traumatizing conditions than those with a higher GABA level (Vaiva *et al.* 2004).

DOES YOGA HELP TRAUMA CLIENTS?

A number of teams of researchers studying subjects with various types of traumatization have been able to prove that yoga has a positive effect on PTSD symptoms: after natural catastrophes, in the military environment, in complex and sexual traumatization, and in dissociative disorders (Brown and Gerbarg 2009; Carter and Byrne 2004, 2006; Khalsa Dharma Singh and Stauth 2004; Lilly and Hedlund 2010; Sageman 2002, 2004; Stankovic 2011; Telles, Naveen, and Dash 2007; van der Kolk, McFarlane, and Weisaeth 2006).

YOGA AND/OR EXPOSURE THERAPY?

Jennifer Johnston, who studied the impact of yoga on military personnel in her doctoral dissertation, confirmed the positive effect of yoga (2011). All 12 participants in her study experienced a significant reduction in the symptoms surveyed by CAPS (Clinician-Administered PTSD Scale) after a ten-week practice period. This also applied to the extent of overexcitation. According to her study, the use of yoga in trauma therapy is supported by the fact that it did not produce a worsening of the symptoms in any of the cases. Other researchers also confirm Johnston's perspective. On the other hand, there are reports in the literature that other treatments (such as exposure therapy) worsened the symptoms of some veterans. Some warn against a form of treatment that is too one-sided when keeping an eye on more than just the reduction of symptoms. Pitman and colleagues (1991) believe that some people who receive exposure treatment with trauma-related stimuli tend to be retraumatized instead of cured. In these cases, the psychobiological secondary diseases are worsened instead of improved.

This could lead to the following conclusion. For those who cannot tolerate exposure therapy, yoga can represent an effective means of supporting them in their affect regulation and tolerance. Preliminary yoga sessions or a combination of therapeutic interventions would be a blessing for these people.

So does yoga help in better tolerating the strains of exposure therapy? Descilo and his team (2010) provided some interesting information on this topic. They compared the effect of yoga breathing in combination with exposure therapy to that of yoga breathing without therapy. They studied 50 clients who had suffered from PTSD after the 2004 tsunami in Indonesia. They divided the affected people into three groups: (1) yoga breathing, (2) yoga breathing combined with exposure therapy, and (3) on a waiting list. The clients learned breathing techniques. Those in the exposure group 2 additionally received three to five one-on-one sessions with Traumatic Incident Reduction (TIR). As expected, groups 1 and 2 showed significant reductions in PTSD symptoms.

A personal observation by Descilo in the study is especially interesting. He wrote: "However, case studies of clients who had previously been unable to tolerate TIR showed that when yoga breathing preceded TIR, they were then able to tolerate and benefit from TIR." When yoga is offered simultaneously or before the trauma therapy, we can assume that fewer clients would break off the therapy. According to Descilo, clients who were able to tolerate the exposure therapy did not show any better results through the combination of breathing exercises and exposure therapy.

YOGA AND/OR COGNITIVE–VERBAL INTERVENTIONS?

A further study examined the impact of combining yoga and a simple verbal intervention. When studying subjects who had experienced domestic violence, Franzblau *et al.* (2006) linked yoga with disclosure (conversation with a non-judgmental listener), and divided the subjects into four groups for this purpose: (1) yoga group, (2) yoga plus disclosure, (3) just disclosure, and (4) control group. The participants of groups 1–3 evaluated themselves more positively in parameters such as self-efficacy, self-control, security, fear, and trust than before the intervention. Combination group 2 experienced the greatest benefit.

Franzblau *et al.* (2006) draw the following conclusion. Breathing and physical exercises make it easier to gain control over the body and mind, which has a positive impact on fear and depression, reducing these symptoms. All of these findings corroborate the hypothesis that a combination of cognitive with body-related interventions, such as breathing exercises and movement, prove to have synergy effects.

Patricia Gerbarg (2008) described a fascinating development in the treatment for a case of sexual abuse under the inclusion of cognitive–verbal techniques together with body-related techniques (yoga breathing). At the researcher's recommendation, the female client attended a *pranayama* course parallel to conversational therapy, and practiced yoga breathing every day for eight months. During this time, Gerbarg observed considerable progress in the conversational therapy, especially in relation to the client's body image and her panic reactions to men. Gerbarg presumed that the successes in the conversational therapy were based on interoceptive processes through yoga breathing since the messages that provide information about the inner state of the body are constantly sent through the vagus nerve from the body to the interoceptive cortex. This is where they become part of the body image and linked with the emotional reactions, behavior patterns, and decision-making process.

YOGA AND SCHEMA

Much speaks for the impact of yoga primarily occurring on the level of body schema. If the physical sensations are frozen at the time of the trauma, the same information keeps reaching the brain and produces the same feelings, reactions, and sensations there. This frozen trauma information is called "schema." It can prove to be tremendously difficult to find access to the trauma schema just through verbal interventions, as in a conversational therapy. Yet there is the possibility of logging into this interoceptive network and sending therapeutic messages through physical exercises and mental techniques.

The quickest and most effective path is through the breath, since tens of thousands receptors in the lungs and respiratory passages change the messages that are passed on to the brain (Brown and Gerbarg 2009). For example, if we breathe very slowly, the body can send the brain the information that we are safe (Gerbarg 2008).

Because of its synergy effect, yoga can be a meaningful supplement for enduring an exposure therapy. Clients who cannot face processing the burdening traumatic experiences are supported by yoga in developing their affect regulation and resources. The question is whether all of those who were able to go to the exposure would have had less stress if, completely in keeping with the yogic principle of *ahimsa*, they had been given additional tools.

DOES YOGA REPLACE TRAUMA THERAPY?

Bessel van der Kolk, himself a yoga practitioner, is one of the pioneers in the area of integrating the body into trauma therapy. In The Trauma Center at the Justice Resource Institute (JRI) in Brookline, MA, USA, which provides traumatized people with an extensive treatment offer, yoga has become a solid component in the treatment. This is where David Emerson and his team offer TSY for victims of various types of traumas. In their yoga classes they also treat people with complex PTSDs.

In *Trauma-Sensitive Yoga* (Emerson and Hopper 2011; Emerson *et al.* 2009), the yoga teachers place much value on offering variations and choices so that clients get a feeling of control and self-determination. The teachers provide more decisive and differentiated information than is customary in yoga courses about the interoceptive processes in the body to help clients attain a better body awareness. Their formulations are open, leave more leeway for the clients, and are not formulated as instructions.

STUDIES ON THE EFFICACY OF YOGA

At the JRI, van der Kolk and his team conducted a pilot study with 16 women in 2006. One part of the group received a gentle Hatha yoga training, and the other part engaged in Dialectic-Behavioral Therapy (DBT), a group therapy. The changes in symptoms were recorded in self-evaluation questionnaires to measure the PTSD symptoms, positive and negative affects, and body awareness. After eight weeks, the yoga participants showed improvements in all dimensions of the PTSD. These also included a diminishing of negative feelings and an increase in positive feelings. In addition, they reported more vitality and body awareness. Compared with the DBT group, the yoga group even had a greater reduction of symptoms in relation to the frequency and degree of severity. Only the yoga group reported a significant decrease in intrusion frequency, as well as the severity of the hyperarousal, and a pronounced gain in vitality and body awareness (Emerson *et al.* 2009; also described in van der Kolk and Jehuda 2006).

Van der Kolk *et al.*'s most recent randomized study examined the effect of yoga on chronically therapy-resistant PTSD symptoms in 64 women. One half of the group received yoga training and the other half was informed about health issues. The PTSD symptoms, the ability to regulate affects, and depressive and dissociative symptoms improved for both groups. However, the effect was stronger in the yoga group. The especially interesting element of the study results is that the health group experienced a rise in symptoms toward the end of the sessions while the yoga group continued to be stable (van der Kolk *et al.* 2014). On the basis of this result, we can assume that the sense of emotional security in a group can cause a temporary symptom reduction, but does not have a sustainable effect. In the yoga group, just the factor of belonging to the group cannot provide the essential effect.

Personal participant statements from the qualitative interviews that were additionally carried out within the scope of the study may not be scientific evidence for the efficacy, but they provide valuable information about what the women felt. Here are a few examples:

I feel more connected with my body.

I have learned to focus.

I feel stronger and more balanced.

I used to hate my body, but now I am learning to take care of it.

Another study, conducted in Boston in the USA by Jennifer West, also provided hopeful results. She worked with women who had complex traumas, whose complex symptoms could not be treated by exposure therapy alone. She wrote: "Recent conceptualizations of trauma recovery call for a paradigm shift that recognizes not only the need for symptom-reduction, but also the encouragement of positive development and personal growth (i.e. stronger sense of self, relationships with others, and perspective on life)" (West 2011, p.4). Her qualitative study included a ten-week program in which the female subjects attended a trauma-informed Hatha yoga class. The study was related to PTSD symptoms and personal growth (West 2011). Following the training, the participants felt strengthened in six of the studied themes: Gratitude and compassion, Relatedness, Acceptance, Centeredness, and Empowerment (GRACE).

Clients were often unable to "feel" their bodies as their own after trauma. The perception or acknowledgment of their body was "0." Yoga led to 50–60 percent feeling that they had been healed through its practice. One participant remarked on the problem of body control: "I feel like I could be incredibly watchful and if my shoulder went up, I could recognize this it and I'd be like, 'Alright, I can breathe and it will go down'…so, I know that if I do A, that B will eventually happen." Others said that since practicing Yoga they were able to observe what happened in their bodies and were able to change a posture or a breathing pattern; they no longer felt stuck and frozen.

Concerning emotions, some perceived changes such as being able to tolerate affects much better. Yoga helped them to feel like they didn't have to push their emotions away or suppress them. Some observed that they felt more comfortable when they dared to express emotions like anger.

Studies show that yoga has a positive effect on PTSD symptoms that is comparable with other therapy possibilities. But if we consider the elements of psychological processing, we cannot avoid noticing emotional and cognitive processing is necessary in addition to somatic processing. This cannot be provided by purely body-related trauma work.

TRAUMA-INFORMED YOGA

Like TSY, Trauma-Informed Yoga takes into account the fact that dissociation, hypervigilance, and hyperarousal often show a lack of security and are "standard responses" to strong feelings and physical sensations. It is therefore probable that yoga can bring these types of feelings and therefore reactions to the surface, as well as memories, fears, pain, and sensations that are associated with the trauma.

Such triggers can occur in many situations. Trauma-Informed Yoga therefore suggests that we show the beginner postures at the start of the training, and then slowly progress to the advanced asanas in order to not overwhelm participants. Another recommendation is to offer participants as much security and control as possible by allowing them to choose the way in which they want to perform an *asana*. For example, they can decide whether they want to practice with open or closed eyes. Formulate the learning contents in an inviting way and allow the participants to decide what is best for them at the moment. Give them verbal encouragement to become curious about what is happening within their body. Avoid *asanas* in which they could feel vulnerable—such as opening the legs—as well as physical assistance.

9

WHICH COMPONENTS OF YOGA ARE EFFECTIVE?

As we have seen, the studies did not use specific kinds of yoga or *pranayama*. Instead, various types were employed. This makes it difficult to make a precise statement about which components are the most effective in reducing symptoms in trauma clients. Depending on the teacher and the school, there were different types of main emphasis in the studies. The body-oriented *asana* practice, *pranayama*, or a combination of the two disciplines was used. The *asana* practice was also not uniform. In addition to Hatha yoga and TSY, the rather instructional Iyengar yoga discipline (see under the section *"Asanas* or *pranayama"* below) was taught. While there will not be a conclusive answer in response to the question of "Which components are effective?," the studies contain information about which element can be used to develop a meaningful yoga practice for trauma clients.

THE RHYTHM DOES IT

In the traditional sense, yoga is a rhythmic practicing of the *asanas*. This means that we consciously assume a posture, stay in feeling this *asana* for a moment, mindfully come out of it, and then sense it for another moment before we move on to the next position. This going into it and pausing during the exertion, as well as leaving it again, should be imagined as training for the nervous system. This rhythm requires sympathetic and parasympathetic activations to alternate— like stepping on the gas pedal and then the brakes while driving a car. Practices of exertion with subsequent phases of calmness and relaxation train the autonomic nervous system with every repetition. "A majority of the positive effect results from going through several cycles every time when you practice" (Broad 2012, p.149).

According to these considerations, Mayasandra S. Chaya studied more than 100 men to examine the effect of a diverse Hatha yoga routine that trained both the metabolic brake and the gas pedal. Measurements of the respiratory gases showed that the metabolic rate decreased by an average of 13 percent. This up and down appears to generate an inner flexibility, giving the body and mind an opportunity to relax (Broad 2012).

This means that a yoga practice in which sympathetic activation alternates through controlling exertion with a parasympathetic phase of tracing the feelings and calmness is meaningful. Due to its influence on the depth and frequency of breathing, this training also influences the nervous system. If we do yoga in this way, we alternate between stepping on the gas pedal and the brake. In contrast to the customary workout in which a long acceleration phase is followed by an extensive phase of putting on the brakes, this occurs a number of times per hour in shorter intervals in yoga.

According to Swami Satyananda Saraswati:

> After the second or third exercise, sit in the basic posture, close your eyes, and direct your perception to the natural breath, the parts of the body that have just been moved, and all of the arising thoughts or feelings. After about one minute, continue the exercise. This helps not only the body to take a break but also the mind and inner energy patterns that set the spiritual and emotional processes in motion. The relaxation phase is just as important as the *asanas* themselves and must not be skipped. (Saraswati 2010, p.24)

Even if a full minute break is certain to overwhelm trauma clients at the start, it becomes clear that the yogi was always aware of how valuable the starting up and calming down of the nervous system is.

Salmon *et al.* (2004) include an additional aspect of rhythm. They hypothesize that yoga and other repetitive movement patterns train the rhythm of the biological functions, which are interrupted by stress in many cases. The rhythmic movements performed together with others also give practitioners a feeling of relatedness. Berrol (1992) assumes that individuals experience themselves as part of the whole through the synchronous movements. In the therapy practice, a sense of belonging can arise when practicing together.

THE BREATH DOES IT

By simply observing and feeling, the yoga masters have found out that conscious breath control—*pranayama*—can influence the practitioner's mental state. We also immediately sense the effect of various *pranayama* exercises. Breathing at a lower frequency calms and stimulates the ventrovagal parasympathetic part of the nervous system. In contrast, a faster breathing rhythm makes us more alert, but sometimes also nervous and restless. This indicates an activation of the sympathetic nervous system. Many research teams have confirmed this yogic empirical knowledge (Bernardi *et al.* 2001; Bhargava, Gogate, and Mascarenhas 1988; Telles *et al.* 2004, Telles, Singh, and Balkrishna 2011). Fast breathing improves concentration, attention, reaction time, sensomotoric performance, and visual scanning (Telles and Desiraju 1992). On the other hand, slow breathing reduces psychological and physiological stress during fear (Cappo and Holmes 1984).

The first known study on breath control was conducted in the 1930s by Behanan (1937). According to his observations, deep breathing (*Ujjayi* Breath—breathing against resistance, see Chapter 14) causes a delay of mental functions. But at the same time, a state of deep relaxation, inner joy, and a serene, pleasant mood arise. A good 70 years later, Brown and Gerberg (2009) confirmed these results. They found an intensified parasympathetic vagal activation in the practitioners of *Ujjayi* Breath, and associated this effect with various mechanisms: slow breathing, breathing against resistance, holding the breath, and prolonged exhalation. In addition, slow yoga breathing against resistance produces an increase of the alpha waves in the brain, which is associated with a state of relaxation. Furthermore, there is an increase in coherence and synchronicity, which improves neuronal plasticity and learning (Larsen *et al.* 2006).

Another research team studied the effect of the breath in an even more differentiated manner, and compared the normal prolonged exhale with *Ujjayi* Breath. They came up with an interesting result. Although the prolonged exhale increases the parasympathetic activity, *Ujjayi* Breath further improves this effect through more afferent input in the brain. In contrast to the prolonged exhale, it also improves the heart rate variability (HRV) (Telles and Desiraju 1991).

The Bee Breath (*Bhramari Breath*) (exhaling with a humming tone) represents another possibility for influencing the breath. One study investigated its impact on anxiety disorders. After eight weeks, those who had practiced the Bee Breath, singing the "OM" mantra, and the Alternating Breath (alternately breathing through the right and left nostril), reported a decrease in anxiety symptoms. Beyond the subjective results, further evidence is a decreased pulse rate and decline in the metabolic products of adrenaline and noradrenaline, as well as an effect on the physiological processes that suggest parasympathetic activation (Crisan 1984, cited in Telles and Naveen 2008). The measurement of gamma waves resulted in further "proof." Practicing the Bee Breath let these brainwaves suddenly skyrocket. The researchers interpreted this effect as a possible neuronal correspondence with a mental state that accompanies yoga and meditation (Telles and Naveen 2008).

Another classic *pranayama* technique is the Alternating Breath. This way of breathing increases HRV during the practice. In addition, it further slows down the breath rhythm even beyond the practice time (Jovanov 2005).

Since the breathing exercises have a direct influence on the nervous system, they can develop a calming effect. They provide valuable services for trauma clients as a supplement to the *asanas*. In case of an emergency, they can tone down an arousal. When practiced on a regular basis, they provide relaxation and recuperation.

ASANAS OR *PRANAYAMA*?

Many studies do not include precise details on the focus of the practice—*asanas* or *pranayama*—and therefore thwart a differentiated statement on the effect mechanisms. Fortunately, this gap has been closed by two studies examining the effect of a six-week Iyengar yoga training for Vietnam War veterans. The depressive symptoms diminished for the participants, but not their easily inflammable feelings of anger and annoyance or their sleep disorders. When the research team included *Ujjayi* Breath and meditation with this training in a further study, the result was a reduction in both the feelings of anger and sleep disorders (Carter and Byrne 2004).

Iyengar yoga is especially well suited for studies since it has much structure and is performed precisely. People have quite a precise idea of what they get, which isn't always the case for other types of yoga. Iyengar yoga is a type of yoga that is exclusively based on physical training. If the practitioner's own strength or flexibility isn't enough for precisely performing the *asanas*, they work with aids such as blocks or ropes. Practitioners sometimes stay in one posture for quite a long time while another practitioner or the teacher corrects with the aids or is even hands on. The correct form is important!

A later study by the same researcher team showed the following results. The Iyengar yoga positions clearly reduced the depressive symptoms, and the breathing exercises in particular had a significantly positive effect on the PTSD symptoms. Carter and Byrne (2006) presume that the improvements occurred due to various factors such as distraction, self-empowerment, mastering/ability, social interaction, and aerobic physical effort. They also consider it possible that the positions may alleviate depression (for example, *asanas* in which people sit up straight, strengthening *asanas*, and backbends; author's note) will improve the mood, at least for the short term; the breathing exercises and *savasana* (relaxation position while lying down) positively influence sleep disorders, and the more calming positions (such as forward bends and resting positions; author's note) helped them better cope with annoyance (Carter and Byrne 2006).

It is interesting to note that the principles and practices of Iyengar yoga are diametrically opposed to those of TSY. But soldiers, who are accustomed to the drill, may react differently to a type of yoga that strives for the correct form through aids than those who have become traumatized in civilian life. The experience of an abused child or woman who has been raped cannot be equated with the experience of a soldier in battle—even if the consequential symptoms are similar. It is possible that the various target groups need different therapy approaches.

MINDFULNESS AS AN EFFECT FACTOR

For many centuries, mystics of various cultures have practiced meditation with the goal of self-perception, consciousness expansion, and healing (Engel 1999). Both the general and scientific interests in these practices for the development and recuperation of the mind have increased strongly over the past decades (Walsh and Shapiro 2006).

The positive influences of mindfulness on self-healing (Santorelli 1999), acts of self-mutilation (Daubenheimer 2005), chronic worries and brooding (Delgado *et al.* 2010), and the general sense of wellbeing (Brown and Ryan 2003; Brown, Ryan, and Creswell 2007) have been proven many times over. This scientific focus is primarily on changes in the brain of those who meditate. Jha, Krompinger, and Baime (2007) have shown that those who meditate on a regular basis show better executive attention control (conflict monitoring) after the mindfulness training than those who do not meditate. This was already evident in the first measuring result. Conflict monitoring contains mechanisms for the monitoring and mastering of conflicts between thoughts, feelings, and behavior responses.

In the mid-1980s, Merzenich *et al.* (1987) had demonstrated how important concentrated attention is for learning new abilities and ways of behavior. In an experiment with monkeys, the fingers of the animals were stimulated with a drilled dial in which the rhythm occasionally changed. Merzenich could prove that all of those that were rewarded because they did the tactile exercise in a concentrated way and responded to the stimuli variations showed tangible changes in the brain areas responsible for touch stimuli. Those without a reward did not show these changes, even though the stimulus was the same (Perlmutter and Villoldo 2011). According to Merzenich: "Experience coupled with attention leads to physical changes in the structure and future functioning of the nervous system" (cited in Begley 2010, p.159). So if people are entirely involved in something, the brain can locate information. But if they allow themselves to be distracted, a large number of other synaptic circuits are activated. This can dissipate the actual intention. If focused attention is lacking, no new links are made (Dispenza 2009). This means that every task carried out without mindful awareness does not bring any new learning.

The components of the executive attention control were correlated with the activation of the anterior cingulate cortex and the lateral prefrontal cortex (Cahn and Polich 2006; Posner and Rothbart 2007), the brain areas that are also typically activated during meditation. The presumption is that in addition to the effects of meditation on the attention function, the meditation practice trains the regulation of emotions (Ekman *et al.* 2005; Goleman 2003). When compared to non-meditating people, those practicing mindfulness meditation actually show a more quickly decreasing physiological reaction (electrodermal activity) to aversive stimuli, and a reduced modulation of the startle reaction through aversive stimuli (Zeidler 2007). This can be evaluated as a change in the regulation of emotions.

The role of the hippocampus for meditation is also emphasized (Newberg and Iversen 2003). It causes a cortical activation and, in interaction with the amygdala, modulates attention and emotion (Joseph 1996). The activation in the hippocampal regions has been confirmed in various meditation studies (Lazar *et al.* 2005). Since there was repeated proof of a reduced hippocampus volume in trauma clients, which was associated with difficulties in the regulation of emotion, they could benefit from mindfulness practice.

In 2009, an interesting study by Claudia Catani and her team compared the effect of meditation and relaxation techniques with the application of KIDNET, a special form of narrative therapy that was developed for children. The results showed that both KIDNET and meditation and relaxation techniques achieved a comparable decrease in the PTSD symptoms of the 31 participating children. This could still be demonstrated six months later in a follow-up study. The study permits the conclusion that learning a meditation technique has the same effect for children after a natural catastrophe as treatment with a narrative technique.

This result was in contradiction to the research results for the treatment of traumatized adults. In this group, a trauma-focused approach that contained the trauma exposure also resulted in clear benefits—even directly after the event. Consequently, children appeared to respond differently to the treatment possibilities from adults, as the latter probably require cognitive processing and integration.

SUMMARY AND CONCLUSIONS

As clearly explained above, yoga and meditation are not a universal remedy, although they serve us well due to their synergy effects. The treatment of choice appears to be a comprehensive trauma therapy that includes not only the somatic but also the emotional and cognitive processing of traumatic memories. At any rate, this applies to adults.

What does this mean for the use of yoga in trauma therapy? To begin with, there are some fundamental insights that have been established. Due to the research findings, we can assume the following:

- Yoga has a positive effect on stress and the symptoms of simple and complex PTSDs.

- The ability to stay with an exposure therapy is improved when combined with yoga.

- The combination of cognitive with body-related interventions, such as breath training and movement, has synergy effects.

- In addition to symptom reduction, yoga shows further benefits such as improving the general sense of wellbeing and state of the person's health.

- Through its postures and breathing exercises, yoga makes it possible to send therapeutic messages on the interoceptive level that cannot be accessed through verbal techniques.

- Yoga causes structural changes in the brain.

- Yoga has positive effects on the release of neurotransmitters and catecholamines (such as dopamine, noradrenaline, and adrenaline).

- If the exposure therapy is tolerated and can be used successfully, the addition of yoga does not show any improvement in symptoms, but when the general state of health and sense of wellbeing are taken into consideration, yoga can well represent relief for clients, since it has a positive effect on the processing of stress. As a result, it has a holistic effect on the physical and emotional sense of wellbeing.

- It is advantageous to tailor the way in which we use bodywork in the therapy to the needs of people with complex traumas. This means offering a setting with much flexibility and possibilities for creativity.

- People who cannot tolerate an exposure therapy can be helped by yoga in their affect tolerance. As a possibility for improving the ability to regulate affects at the start of the therapy or in a combination of trauma- and body-therapeutic interventions, yoga is beneficial for such people.

- In combination with verbal/cognitive techniques, yoga can have a synergy effect on feelings such as self-efficacy, self-control, and security. These are important therapy goals, especially for clients who have suffered from complex traumatization.

- Yoga can be successfully applied in cases where verbal interventions do not show any effect. Because yoga changes the bottom-up body schemata and breathing patterns, both the affect regulation can be improved and the negative cognitions changed.

- Rhythmic instructions, which alternately train the sympathetic and parasympathetic nervous system, appear to be an advantage. By pausing and sensing/feeling what is happening inside after one or more series of *asanas*, "putting on the brakes" is practiced. With the help of activating/calming *asanas* and breathing exercises, participants learn to influence their nervous system and sense of wellbeing.

- Practicing together promises to create a sense of relatedness, which had previously often been interrupted by stress.

- The choice of positions and breathing exercises can be oriented on the client's degree and type of activation. Sympathetic activation requires different interventions than a dorsal–vagal activation. So *asanas* are offered that tend to be more activating or calming. Each *asana* is subsequently examined in terms of its effectiveness.

- The main focus of the yoga on offer—*asanas* or *pranayama*—can be adapted to the symptoms. But since the symptoms are complex in most cases, the recommended approach is to include both components and adapt them to the emphasis of the main symptoms.

- Movement, and therefore the activation of the sympathetic nervous system, is more effective for depression and dissociation than quiet sitting and breathing.

- Including breathing exercises such as *Ujjayi* Breath and Alternating Breath in the program appears to be advisable since they result in a parasympathetic vagal activation and improve the HRV. They also have a positive effect on sleep disorders and arousal.

- Mindfulness appears to be an essential effect factor since people cannot learn anything new without focusing their attention.

- Mindfulness appears to improve the training of executive attention control, as well improving the ability for conflict monitoring and regulation of emotions.

- Sports such as walking have less intensive effects on the release of calming GABA. This could be related to the effective factor of "mindfulness" or "rhythm."

During my research I repeatedly asked why Iyengar yoga and even other types of yoga that are sometimes very different from a trauma-sensitive approach also take effect and achieve positive results. I do not have a conclusive answer to this. However, I can imagine that war veterans—and many studies have been conducted with this target group—are different from others who are traumatized. They are accustomed to a military drill and were traumatized in a situation that is intensely different from that of a woman who has been raped or an abused child. War veterans "end" their traumatization frequently in a fight mode. They go to war, fight, and therefore do not feel like a victim *per se* or helplessly at the mercy of a situation. In their traumatization, women and children often cannot use fight or flight as possible defensive strategies—the biological way out of the hopeless situation is shutting down. In contrast to the first target group, they have a much greater need to relearn that they have possibilities of control and choice available to them.

The TSY approach, with its focus on self-determination, benefits all traumatized individuals, but especially those who cannot tolerate "normal" yoga (at least not yet). There are no studies that compare the various types of yoga with each other or with the various target groups, so this is still only speculation. Further research may provide us with more clarity in this regard.

The interesting and convincing study results on the positive effect of yoga for PTSD clients have one disadvantage: Without exception, they are based on the practice of yoga in a group setting. Since not every therapist wants to lead groups, the main question is, how can yoga be integrated into trauma therapy and/or the therapy setting?

PART IV

HOW DOES YOGA BECOME PART OF TRAUMA THERAPY?

10

THE METHOD

All of the studies cited in this book report on successes in clients who participated in yoga *groups*, but since my main emphasis is on individual therapy, the question arises as to how experiences from the studies can flow into the therapeutic practice.

This is the first thought to keep in mind: No matter with which therapy concept you treat clients with complex PTSDs, certain preconditions basically need to be fulfilled (cf. Wöller 2006).

BASIC REQUIREMENTS FOR TRAUMA THERAPY

SECURITY

A main principle is that the design of the surroundings and relationship must offer a "maximum contrast to traumatic situations." The following points are essential in this context. A traumatic experience is frequently characterized by disrespect for the affected person and their needs. It is intrinsically associated with insecurity. Our task is to perceive and value the client's needs, as well as recognizing that these needs are legitimate. This gradually allows a feeling of inner security to develop. The greatest security factor in practicing yoga is that there are no errors. We offer a relationship on an equal footing and are interested in the client's experiences, which we never judge.

CONTROL

In significantly traumatic situations, trauma clients experience a loss of control. We therefore provide them with a maximum of control. We encourage them to see our recommendations and advice as offers, examine the interventions in terms of their success, and reject or modify interventions that are not very helpful. Every *asana* and *pranayama* is an invitation and simultaneously guidance for clients to regain control. The clients determine whether and in which way they want to follow our recommendations. The precondition for this is that we have choices and alternatives to offer.

Our initial responsibility is to create a balance between closeness and distance. We also signal through our presence that we are "there," and do not demand or judge anything. Real presence requires our attention and vigilance.

ATTAINING DISTANCE FROM AFFECTS

The ability to regulate the intensity of affects is just as weakened in our clients as their ability to focus attention. Being in touch with the emotions caused by trauma, they frequently perceive undifferentiated affective states with diffuse and unbearable tension. Traumatized people are usually unable to immediately respond to emotion-triggering stimuli, but are flooded by emotions shortly thereafter. This high level of arousal lowers the threshold for experiencing intrusions, panic attacks, and dissociative states. A first important step is exploring what has helped clients in the past to deal with their overwhelming emotions. These experiences will be supplemented with exercises from the therapy setting. Making lists will help them to recognize their existing and new possibilities, as well as systematically put them to use.

AFFECT DIFFERENTIATION

Affect differentiation is an important task in psychotherapy with the goal of learning to distinguish between the emotional qualities, to feel each of them separately, and to become able to discern between traumatic and non-traumatic emotional qualities. It is just as important to create boundaries between the origin of the current feeling and this feeling in the past. For clients, both are frequently merged with each other. Once they can separate the two, they experience a sense of relief. It is also important to be able to distinguish between internal and external threats: between the acute danger that demands action and overwhelming, paralyzing traumatic fear. Various affects are often located in different parts of the body and also do not feel the same. This is where we can start with the initial possibilities for differentiation.

RESOURCES

For many clients, access to their own resources is buried. Some have the feeling that they don't have any resources available to them at all. It is useful to have resource techniques that help clients remember the good and powerful moments of their life and to intensively experience them. In short, this means anchoring the resource techniques with a body movement or an object. Asking the clients to imagine inner helper figures that they can ask for support or advice at any time supplements the practice of the safe place to which clients can withdraw in their minds.

Resources such as *asanas* or *pranayama* play a major role in the body-oriented approach. In addition to the imaginative approaches, they make physical *action* possible.

SELF-CARE

The nature of adequate self-care is being able to stand up for our own needs, setting boundaries against other people's demands, trusting in close relationships, protecting ourselves against violent assaults, and regulating closeness and distance. Many traumatized clients experience a generalized helplessness that makes them blind to the idea that they can do something for themselves. They are often convinced that they do not deserve any self-care because they tenaciously cling to the internalized prohibition of caring for themselves. Some also cannot adequately perceive or articulate their needs. Self-hatred and anger directed towards themselves can thwart self-care.

Being gentle with the body, not always going to the limits, and paying attention to vulnerable areas such as the knees or spinal column can be the first steps in the direction of self-care. As therapists, we are role models for this attitude by treating ourselves with gentleness and mindfulness.

ATTACHMENT EXPERIENCE AND MENTALIZATION

Mentalization is understood as the ability to perceive our own mental states and those of others, classifying them as needs, wishes, expectations, and beliefs. This ability for reflection on our own and other people's psychological states is an essential precondition for successful relationships. The ability for mentalization is trained in a secure attachment relationship. Abuse and traumatization restrict the aptitude for self-reflection.

Mentalization primarily depends on the experienced burden of stress and the quality of the emotion regulation. Clients who normally have an adequate mentalization can lose this ability in stress situations. It is typical for traumatized clients to have mature and immature parts existing in parallel. This explains how they are capable of mentalization with the adult part but not with the immature, traumatized child part. Mentalization is correlated with a good functioning of the prefrontal cortex, and also with the anterior cingulate cortex. These are precisely the structures that are damaged through the impact of traumas.

THE ABILITY OF SELF-OBSERVATION AND REFLECTION

Clients often express their thoughts and memories in an abundance of confusing and often contradictory statements, so it helps them to work out a comprehensible sequence of their experiencing and behavior. Through intellectual games, they become more detached and recognize that there is more than just one possibility. Attention is focused on the way in which clients describe their current mental states, the significance that it has for them, under which conditions it developed, and how they are influenced in their reactions by their counterpart or their own expectations and fears.

When clients learn to explore and fantasize about which mental states, motivations, and feelings could have predominated in their counterpart, they begin to think through the situations and can contemplate different courses of action. In addition to thinking things through, the observation of physical sensations can strengthen the ability for self-observation. This is how clients can also create more distance within themselves.

PRINCIPLES FOR A BODY-ORIENTED APPROACH

If we transfer these requirements to a body-oriented therapy setting, we can verbally and non-verbally ensure that traumatized clients have their needs met. The principles of a body-oriented setting under consideration of the above-listed requirements for a successful trauma therapy are explained in the following.

Even though this book's main focus is on the integration of body therapy possibilities in direct contact with clients—since this allows for an individual approach to the triggers and resources—information on the group setting is also provided.

Some general parameters and principles should be observed when working with both groups and individuals. Here is an excerpt of guidelines developed by Lilly and his team (2010):

- Participants feel better with a guided mediation than with silence; silence can frighten them.

- Practitioners should always make their own decision as to whether they keep their eyes open or closed during relaxation, *pranayama*, or performing the *asanas*.

- The light in the room is not switched off or dimmed.

- Avoid physical corrections, except when participants are in danger of seriously injuring themselves. Demonstrate the exercise for them or use verbal correction possibilities.

- Wear normal, non-revealing clothing.

- While you should consider the gender of clinical therapists and yoga teachers, the presence of a male or female instructor or therapist can also have healing components, depending on the perpetrator's gender.

Every yoga position may be a trigger, and this possibility cannot be completely excluded. But there are *asanas* and *pranayama* that act as stronger triggers or hardly have any effect. Here are some examples, which can be added to depending on the target group:

- Holding the breath.

- Very fast breathing such as the Bellows Breath (*Bhastrika* Breath) (see below). These breathing techniques can be useful in getting people out of a parasympathetic shut-down. However, they should only be introduced gradually after clients have practiced the simple breathing exercises.

- Poses in the all-fours position, in which the pelvis is tilted upward (as in Downward Dog Pose) should only be introduced when clients feel safe. Never stand behind clients when they are doing these positions. This principle applies to all of the exercises.

- Poses that focus on the pelvis can often only be shown at a later time—sometimes only after months of practice.

- For victims of war and torture, stretching and extending may remind them of their experiences of torture.

- Being faced with a choice can also trigger traumatic memories in victims of war or torture. In their torture, some of these clients have experienced being forced to choose between two impossible options.

- A break or quiet phase that is too long can also have a frightening effect.

Bellows Breath (*Bhastrika Breath*) is a powerful, forced breathing in which the belly, like a bellows, arches in the front when inhaling and is drawn in while exhaling. Clients usually do not practice more than 5–10 *Bhastrika Breaths* since this unaccustomed breathing pattern can cause dizziness.

Talk about the known triggers with your clients. Introduce new poses or movements by agreeing on them. You should demonstrate them and formulate this as a recommendation. In no case is this about avoiding triggers. However, a cautious approach should be taken in TSY, which applies to trauma therapy in general.

11

POSSIBLE PRACTICE SETTINGS

Depending on our objectives and inclinations as therapists, as well as that of our clients, there are various alternatives for how body-oriented work with yoga can flow into the trauma therapy. First, we can teach yoga in a small group. Introducing yoga as an independent element before or after a therapy session and practicing a personal yoga program with clients is a second option. The sequence can be tailored to the respective needs and goals such as acquiring resources, achieving relaxation, or learning how to stop habitual dissociation. Clients can use the strategies worked out in this way in everyday life. They can also benefit from the therapeutic process since both the therapist and the client can fall back on them. A third path is weaving the yoga exercises into the therapeutic process.

The common factor of all settings is that they create a space for experimenting in which we practice together and have our respective experiences. The main difference between the group or instructional setting and weaving the physical exercises into the therapy process is that a monolog occurs in the first case. We offer instructions, the clients practice with us, and they modify the exercises as they prefer. There are attempts at dialog, but mainly when the suitable exercises are discussed. Interoceptive experiences and effects of the *asanas* and *pranayama* exercises are the predominant contents of the conversation.

But when we weave the exercises into the process support, the experiences are verbalized and made available through language. This exchange allows for the experiences to be available for clarification, reflection, and processing. In every case, the language and our choice of words play a significant role. Consequently, trauma-oriented body therapy is in no way a non-verbal therapy method, since speaking and movement are attuned in many ways.

TRAUMA-SENSITIVE YOGA IN A GROUP SETTING

Clients who often feel fear, shame, and stress when participating in a group can also benefit from the group setting of TSY. The sense of belonging with other people and feeling like part of something bigger are this setting's advantages.

One participant had the following words for this experience:

> Despite the stress in the group setting, I have had the experience of how strongly "doing" things together connects us: being in a safe framework and without the pressure of having to work toward a specific goal. I can't remember ever having felt like I belonged to a group and was accepted. For me, the yoga mat meant a safe ground that showed me what my place is.

However, the following statements by participants in an eight-week course reveal how much courage is necessary to be part of a yoga group. At the same time, this feedback reveals that the group experience opens up possibilities that we cannot offer in the individual therapy:

> Especially in relation to relaxation and bodywork, I sometimes have a bit of difficulty in opening up to or feeling good in a group.

> I still find being in a group stressful. I'm happy when I get a spot at the edge. But this no longer feels so vitally important to me.

> Even though the group is small, I still have a hard time when it comes to relaxing.

> It's great that we can laugh together.

> I'm happy that everyone is busy with themselves, and I don't feel like anyone is watching me—not even the instructor.

> I experienced the other participants as very appreciative.

> Over time, it has become easier for me to be in the group.

TSY groups offer benefits. For example, in the individual therapy, we have recourse to tools that clients have already explored and practiced in the group. On the other hand, participation in a group serves as exposure. For many of my clients, this is the first occasion in a long time that they have gone into a room with a number of people. At the beginning of the yoga session, I discuss what the focus of my instructions will be. This topic may be the breath, movement, muscle strength, or relaxation. During the hour, I remind them of this focus time and again.

The *asanas* and *pranayama* learned in the group are just as beneficial in the individual therapy as the experiences that clients have had in the group and bring into the therapy session with them. I separate the yoga group and therapy in as far as the groups do not have any beginning, concluding, or mental state rounds. When we do yoga together, I like to leave the focus on the physical experiencing and not bring the clients back to the cognitive level by having them verbalize something. The experience is personal and allowed to remain just that.

If you decide to instruct a group, first practice the program for yourself, and get feedback in your intervision or supervision group. I found it a great help to film myself while practicing, observing both my physical and verbal forms of expression. This allows me to make any necessary corrections. When we try out and vary the *asanas* by ourselves, we can train our own interoception, speaking skills, and yoga voice.

If we put together a program for a group, we are not relying on variety but a sense of security and reliability. We continue to follow the same procedure. A familiar sequence gives people a sense of security and routine. We can introduce variations and increase the degree of difficulty. Once we see that the clients feel secure enough, we can invite them to try out something new. However, we should not introduce more than one or two new *asanas* per hour but explain why we do not constantly change the sequence. We also cannot emphasize often enough that this is not about a perfect position or the correct performance of the *asanas*. Instead, the goal is for clients to once again feel their own body, and the best way to achieve this is by always doing the same *asanas* or breath exercises, attentively observing how our *experiences* vary and change.

A POSSIBLE SEQUENCE FOR A 50-MINUTE GROUP SESSION

The following suggestion is intended to provide an idea of how a group program could be structured. The phase of noticing sensations and pausing that follows after every exercise is not explicitly mentioned each time. It is the basis for experiencing "safe" relaxation.

SEATED POSES

- Seated Mountain Pose—grounding
- Being aware of our breathing
- Head circles and/or moving to the right and left
- Circle or loosen shoulders
- Torso circles
- Side bend right/left
- Cat–Cow with breath synchronization
- Transition to standing

STANDING POSES

- Mountain Pose standing up
- Dynamic side bend right/left
- Downward Dog (possibly with the help of a chair)
- Three-Legged Dog (possibly with the help of a chair)
- Forward bend in standing, back-and-forth movements or "yes/no" head movements
- Warrior I or II Pose
- Mountain Pose with Sun Breath

SEATED POSES

- Seated Mountain Pose—grounding
- Triangle right/left

- Knees to chest

- Seated relaxation

- Bee Breath or Alternating Breath

I usually offer blocks of between eight to ten meetings for 50 minutes each. In this way, the obligation for those involved remains reasonable and the participation still shows an effect.

PRACTICE RULES FOR TRAUMA-SENSITIVE YOGA GROUPS

Emerson and his team (Emerson and Hopper 2011; Emerson *et al.* 2009; Emerson, 2012) have summarized the principles for leading groups in the following way.

KEY ASPECTS

- Security: The room is quiet and prepared.

- Predictability: Instruction times, facilities, and instructor remain constant.

- Flexibility and adaptability: Clients know that their wishes are taken seriously and that they can make adaptations on their own.

TRAUMA-SENSITIVE YOGA SUBJECTS

- Experiencing the present moment: Clients are able to stay in the here and now.

- Making use of choices: Clients are able to adapt the exercises to their own needs.

- Performing effective actions: Clients allow themselves to do something that makes them feel safer, better, more comfortable, etc.

- Perceiving the rhythm of the body: Through breathing and movement clients learn to experience synchronicity in their own bodies and within the group.

GUIDELINES FOR INSTRUCTORS

- Exercises: A slow, steady pace makes it easier to experience body awareness than faster exercise sequences.

- Language: Tone of voice and choice of words are open and inviting.

- Assistance: Visual corrections and verbal support.

- Surroundings: The instructor is present and compassionate.

FURTHER IMPORTANT POINTS

- For yoga on chairs and while standing, normal clothes can be worn—there is no need for special gym wear.

- Clients may practice with or without shoes.

- If people still wish to get changed, there should be a possibility for doing so discretely.

- The light in the room is normal and not dimmed.

- The room is of an appropriate size, so that the clients don't get into each other's space, regardless of whether they are sitting on a chair or standing.

- The size of the group is kept small. I work with five to six clients.

- The clients are separated according to gender.

- The group leader stays in one place, from where they can instruct the group and let the group know. Clients need be sure that they won't be touched unexpectedly.

TSY groups can turn out to be a challenge for therapists. Here is an example. A female client who attended a group on a regular basis often looked bored, played with her mobile phone, or stared at the ceiling. I became aware of my own tension—I didn't know whether her behavior was because of me or because of the exercises. However, I wanted to follow the premise of free choice and not ask her to participate. To my greatest surprise, she wrote me a card at the end of the course that expressed how much the yoga meant to her and how much she liked coming to it. And she emphasized that she never felt judged or assessed.

Many clients need something that helps them find their way back to themselves when the activity in the group becomes too much for them. If we are serious about freedom in decision-making and a relationship on an equal footing that stands out due to its maximum differentiation from a traumatizing situation, we must learn to tolerate such situations.

Despite all of the challenges in which we can explore our inner attitude and expand our ability for mindfulness, being allowed to participate in the development of each individual—as well as that of a group—is one of the most exhilarating experiences. Lilly and his team (2010), who researched the effect of yoga groups for sexually traumatized people, commented as follows:

> Sharing yoga with young people recovering from sexual abuse has been one of the most satisfying avenues of yoga service the authors have been fortunate to experience. The boys and girls show such a bruised beauty that when the practice begins, it's hard to say how they will respond. But when the sessions start, and they begin to feel safe, truly safe, both inside and out, you can feel the power of yoga. (Lilly *et al.* 2010, p.11)

REPORT BY A TRAUMA-SENSITIVE YOGA GROUP MEMBER

> The starting point for my decision to open up to yoga was becoming aware that I was unable to sense my body, let alone control it or feel good in it. Specific questions in my trauma therapy (such as "Where do you feel something? Do you sense your arms? Your legs?") allowed me to recognize that I apparently lacked this basic ability so familiar to everyone else. "How can you sense your body?" This question, as well as the perception that I couldn't do this, caused me severe despair. I could hardly tolerate my inadequacy. On the other hand, did I really want to feel this hated body?! But I understood that this was imperative if I wanted to change the inadequate quality of my life and the missing sense of security within and with myself.
>
> At the first yoga session, I arrived late through no fault of my own and without clothes for yoga. This had the negative consequence for

me that the yoga mats were already "taken" by those who had arrived on time. The only one left was in the middle. Great! It was my own fault. Help!

In the following sessions, my therapist made sure that I could unroll my mat behind those of the others, where I felt safer. So she was the only person who could see me—none of the other participants could. This made it possible for me to start opening up at all, and getting somewhat accustomed to the situation.

The first sessions were mainly stressful for me: not attracting too much attention, being able to keep up, seeming "normal"…and just not feeling myself. As long as I can remember, it has always been difficult for me to confront my body. Having to look at or touch its individual areas was an anxiety-provoking challenge. Often enough, I started these yoga sessions in dissociative states or was paralyzed by old memories.

I was surprised that it was possible to keep the fear at bay when I could concentrate on a yoga position or a breath rhythm. Sometimes I even forgot that I was afraid! But if the absence of fear wasn't the same as courage, was it perhaps a sense of safety??? It actually was. These were my first cautious experiences that I could feel safe in a group, but ultimately also with myself, or could at least experience moments without fear. Finding yourself outside of the relationship level and far from demands of specifically having to achieve something represented trying out possibilities for me. So it was something that I could succeed at and also gave me a sense of security. Step by step, I succeeded in reducing fears and developing the sense of security— and even did this within a group! However, the yoga sessions in the group remained something that I mainly tried to tolerate for quite some time; the changes only developed gradually.

The instructions on the *asanas* and *pranayamas* were straightforward, so practicing became feasible for me. These were little successes with much significance for my nervous system. First, I could do something. Second, this experience of success was repeated by each individual *asana*. I noticed bit by bit that I no longer felt paralyzed at the end of the yoga sessions, that the pull of the trauma in my head and body had faded or at least become much weaker, and that I could even go home with a sense of my body. I hadn't known this before. With the bodywork, many more changes were possible than with cognitive work. On top of this, it was the beginning of a differentiated perception of my inner experiencing.

TRAUMA-SENSITIVE YOGA AT THE BEGINNING AND/OR END OF A THERAPY SESSION

Especially at the beginning of the trauma therapy I usually experience what a heroic act it is for some clients to come to the practice, and how good the first contact can be for becoming "able to work." Here is an example to briefly explain what this can look like.

CASE EXAMPLE: KATE

Kate was always nervous when she came to the session. She had cold, sweaty hands, and was very pale. Since we had already worked with *asanas* and *pranayama*, I suggested that we start the session this time with some *asanas* standing up. These could ground her, providing her with a bit more balance and stability. After we had initially gotten into standing Mountain Pose and added some extension and stretching exercises, side bends, etc. to it, she said: "It's better, but I still don't feel like I'm really here." So I suggested that we get into Tree Pose. She was very unsteady and constantly had to try to balance herself (she was normally quite stable when standing in Tree Pose). After changing to the other leg and returning to Mountain Pose, she said: "I just noticed how much I've gotten out of balance, but now I'm back again." We added Powerful Pose and a Warrior Pose so that she felt even more of her own strength. Then we sat down to explore what had thrown her off balance.

For clients who tend to be in a rather dissociative state, good possibilities for ending the dissociation through muscle activity are— as described above—Tree Pose, Downward Dog, Warrior variations, or even Staff Pose or Powerful Pose on a chair. I prefer standing poses since the change of setting and perspective (I am taller when I stand) can curb the regression. However, the choice always depends on what clients experience as conducive.

Starting or ending the therapy session with *pranayama* can become a ritual for some clients so that things don't "start right away" or they "don't have to quickly readjust to everyday life." This creates a type of buffer zone that allows time for arriving or getting ready to leave. Clients often experience this type of deceleration as very soothing. For example, this is the case when they are activated as they arrive at the session, and the arousal can be calmed through familiar and effective breathing exercises. They get a strong feeling of empowerment. Clients also have the experience that even little arousals are worth paying attention to before they become big waves.

Once they have discovered which breath variations are calming for them, these can represent a transition at the end of the session. For example, hyperarousal resulting from an exposure can be mitigated through *pranayama* techniques. The same thing obviously also applies when clients are in a dissociated state. However, my experience has been that the activating power of the *asanas* is more efficient here. In every case, all of this should be tried out and attuned to the needs of clients!

When I practice the yoga *asanas* and *pranayama* with clients, we move to a different place: I have special seating arrangements for yoga, which means that we consciously change the location. I do not want to mix the therapeutic conversation with the practice of yoga *asanas* and *pranayama*. The chairs are not placed directly across from each other but somewhat offset so that we do not sit in a confrontational way. I make sure that there is enough space. I leave it up to the clients to take off their shoes or keep them on, and I do the same as them. I work in street clothes and only offer exercises that can be done without getting changed. Changing their clothes or taking some of them off can be a trigger for some clients. I want to switch as spontaneously as possible from the therapy armchair to yoga. This is why this book only contains exercises that fulfill these preconditions.

FEEDBACK FROM A FEMALE CLIENT IN AN INDIVIDUAL SETTING

My therapist's suggestion to include my body in the therapy left me surprised and also overwhelmed. But I also noticed that I was "often no longer present" in the therapy sessions and was still imprisoned afterward in the feelings and topics that we discussed. The (old) sense of helplessness from the traumatization—the feeling of having failed and being incapable—often remained at the end.

We agreed to do 20 minutes of yoga together after each therapy session—as an experiment. Feeling the therapist's undivided attention during the yoga sessions was difficult for me at the start. It helped me to not have her sitting frontally across from me. Instead, she moved her mat more to the side. This meant that her straight field of vision faced the wall. She didn't look directly at me, which relieved much of my tension and thoughts of running away. Her encouraging feedback had a positive effect on my tension. The feeling that I could do something to reduce my tension helped me, as did discovering and tolerating the body perceptions that had been unfamiliar to me up to that time. The pull in my muscles during the stretching exercises and having more space in my body and greater ease when inhaling after intensive breathing exercises—all of this felt like coming home after being gone for many years.

Despite everything, even the smallest moments of success were still accomplishments! Being capable of doing something—whether a pose or bodily perception—meant power and control. Powerful instead of powerless. Feeling alive instead of paralyzed. Pride and joy instead of depression. The successes motivated and strengthened me. The fears decreased in both their frequency and intensity. Tension gave way to relaxation. The focus was on discovering and trying out things, and there were no pre-defined goals that had to be achieved. So failure was no longer possible, and this relief meant a new experience! The yoga training ended the trauma memories from the therapy session and took away the oppressive burden of the trauma chaos. And yoga considerably reduced my sleep disorders.

What have I learned? For PTSD clients, blockages in experiencing and adequate actions cannot be resolved with just the intellect alone. Having an understanding for themselves, comprehending what happened in the past—as well as what this experience has triggered and destroyed—is undoubtedly important and valuable. But these perceptions still do not make it possible to build a bridge to the body. It remains inaccessible, uncontrollable, and unreliable. The body-centered work built this bridge, which connects the mind with the body.

Because I had been involved in track and field in the past, training my body was not foreign to me. But I never really felt good during or after the training. The focus was on the pressure to succeed. Mindfulness, care, and consideration of my own experiencing were alien concepts. Drill and the ability to adapt were required and encouraged my PTSD symptoms more than providing something to counteract them. The offer of simply exploring and experiencing yoga as an individual possibility ultimately allowed me to discover my *self* in a form that I had been completely unaware of.

PLANNING AND DEVELOPING A YOGA PROGRAM

After we have experienced the various *asanas* and *pranayama* techniques, it is often helpful for clients to have this training written down as a program. We usually start with the first exercises such as feeling the feet, getting into Mountain Pose, or practicing a calming breathing technique. If these elements of the session were helpful, they can be used at home—and this creates a kind of mini-program. When further effective elements are added, we take the time to include them in a process that clients can make into their own. I draw the exercise instructions in the form of stick figures and add the corresponding comments so that clients can also master them, even in difficult moments—it's easier to comprehend an image than text when stressed.

Depending on whether clients tend toward dissociation and need more activating exercises or recommendations against hyperarousal, we work out the corresponding training. The processes are individual and oriented upon the experiences in the therapy session. However, I would still like to provide examples of a more activating and a more calming program.

AN EXAMPLE OF AN ACTIVATING PROGRAM WHILE SEATED

- Seated Mountain Pose as the starting position
- Side bend with change of sides, coordinated with breathing and strong movement
- Triangle with strong breathing
- 3–5 strengthening Bellows Breaths, break; possibly repeat
- Staff Pose, move each leg up and down and coordinate with breath

- Powerful Pose, little movements downward and upward, again in the breathing rhythm

- Seated Mountain Pose, noticing sensations

AN EXAMPLE OF A SEQUENCE FOR ACTIVATION IN STANDING

- Standing Mountain Pose as starting position

- Side bend with change of sides, coordinated with breathing and strong movement

- Warrior I or II, right/left

- Downward Dog Pose

- Three-Legged Dog Pose, alternating right and left leg

- 3–5 strong Bellows Breaths, break; possibly repeat

- Mountain Pose as conclusion

Asanas that synchronize breathing and movement prevent clients from holding their breath. If we would like to avoid having clients hold their breath in a powerful posture while practicing at home—this often happens entirely automatically—we can advise them to mentally count the breaths and decide for how many breaths they want to stay in one *asana*. Counting the breaths reminds them to also let the breath flow when they exert themselves. As an alternative, they can use the right thumb to touch the fingertips of the right index finger, middle finger, ring finger, and little finger and count from 1 to 4 as they do so (index finger 1, middle finger 2, etc.). Then continue counting to 8 with the left hand.

The sense of movement can also be trained when the poses are consciously and mindfully assumed and released again. This is why I always emphasize the sequence of movements when getting into an *asana*.

When overexcitation prevails—which is a sympathetic activation—I tend to offer seated positions and breathing exercises. Grounding exercises, forward bends, the Sun Breath, and Mountain Pose can be meaningful, but always provided that these poses have already been tried out and do not represent triggers. A couple of selected *asanas* and *pranayama* exercises can support clients in stepping on the brakes.

AN EXAMPLE OF A CALMING SEQUENCE SITTING DOWN

- Starting position: Seated Mountain Pose
- Feel the feet and sense the sitting bones—contact with the floor or the seat
- Gentle torso circles
- Bee Breath or Alternating Breath
- Cat–Cow movements with synchronized breath
- Forward bends
- Mountain Pose as the conclusion

A rhythm emerges in each of the sample sequences in that pausing and noticing sensations are always included. However, we can also quite deliberately offer a rhythmic sequence that clients can practice at home (see below).

AN EXAMPLE OF A RHYTHMIC PRACTICE SEQUENCE

- Seated Mountain Pose as the starting position
- 5–10 *Ujjayi* Breaths—parasympathetic nervous system
- 5 Bellows Breaths—sympathetic nervous system
- Make contact with the floor or the seat—parasympathetic nervous system
- Staff Pose, alternating raising and lowering of right and left leg, synchronized breath—sympathetic nervous system
- Gentle Cat–Cow movements with synchronized breath—parasympathetic nervous system

on the objective, this can lead away from the pull of the trauma to the resources or, when there is already more stability, support clients in exploring a distressing experience. In Part VI there are extensive examples of how body-related work finds its place in the therapy process, and how to precisely follow therapeutic goals.

PLANNING THE THERAPY

Yoga cannot and should not replace trauma therapy. Instead, it represents a possibility for supporting clients in tolerating an exposure therapy. If the synergy effects are used, both the therapist and the client will benefit equally. A stabilization phase—in which the relationship is developed and clients should become more stable through exercises—is normally planned for this purpose. If we offer body-related tools to clients for affect regulation, this often gives them a sense of stability since they feel that they have something to help them counteract the pull of the trauma. At the same time, this solidifies the relationship between therapist and client, because trust generally increases when people feel that they are taken seriously and offered concrete effective help.

How can yoga find its place in therapy planning? I would first like to point out that I do not consider stabilizing yoga exercises to be a basic prerequisite for successful trauma therapy. If a client is capable of mastering the exposure therapy, we can and should start this as soon as possible. Through delay and mutual avoidance, we create neither self-trust nor trust in a relationship and increase the suffering.

A few specific exercises that are worked out together always offer an advantage—they make it easier for the clients. They can fall back on them when the stress becomes too intense—both during the therapy session and outside of it. However, I would like to remind you at this point that yoga *asanas* and *pranayama* are not just stabilization tools; they serve equally well in the exposure of somatic triggers.

If we now look at the different setting variations, this gives us various possibilities for how yoga exercises can be considered in the planning of a trauma therapy.

TRAUMA-SENSITIVE YOGA IN THE GROUP

If you have the opportunity of offering a yoga group parallel to the trauma therapy, I recommend that you point out this option to your clients at the beginning of the therapy, and obviously also during the exposure therapy. In the group, clients can become familiar with the *asanas* and *pranayama* exercises that benefit them in the distressing phase of the exposure. They can also fall back on them to mitigate arousals or end dissociation more quickly. After having finished the exposure therapy, clients are are free to decide whether they want to attend a "normal" yoga class, stop practicing, or continue to come to the group. The length of group participation is oriented upon the progress of competence in affect regulation and the client's wishes.

TRAUMA-SENSITIVE YOGA BEFORE AND/ OR AFTER A THERAPY SESSION

If there is no opportunity of attending a course, the practice of *asanas* and *pranayama* can also take place within the therapy session. I begin at the start of the therapy—during the psychoeducation—with the first exercises and instructions. During this phase, the yoga part can take up between one-third to one-half of the therapy session. As a rule of thumb, the bodywork in the first five to ten sessions could take between 15 and 30 minutes. As clients achieve an improved affect tolerance, this time period can be successively reduced since they can then use the resources worked out in this way on their own. If necessary, clients can also be reminded of the repertory that has been worked out and fall back on it in the therapy. How this phase of the therapy is designed depends very much on the client's history. If they have very few resources, more than ten sessions in which the focus must be on affect regulation could be necessary. If possible, I offer double sessions at the start of the therapy, so that there is enough time for the therapeutic conversation after practicing a yoga program. Here is a brief example from my practice, which is intended to illustrate this aspect.

CASE EXAMPLE: FEMALE CLIENT

A 19-year-old female client consulted me after a hospital stay due to depression and self-injuring behavior. She had been sexually abused by various relatives for many years, and now wanted to start a trauma therapy. At the first meeting, she sat across from me in a total state of tension. Her hands and legs were literally intertwined with each other. My first attempts to coax her out of this position with gentle movements failed miserably since she felt a dramatic rise in her arousal during even the slightest relaxing of the tension. After that, I suggested that she try a few strengthening, strenuous poses: Warrior I, Warrior II, and Powerful Pose. Her arousal, which she had never described as less than 4 on a scale of 1–10, went down to "2"—to her astonishment.

So we started the next therapy sessions with strengthening *asanas* in which she felt strong. Afterward, we switched to the therapeutic conversation and finished each session with strengthening *asanas*. The urge to hurt herself after a therapy session gradually diminished, and we were able to turn to her traumatic memories after eight sessions. The yoga *asanas* accompanied us for another eight sessions, but they became less essential and we only resorted to them at the end of the sessions or in case of an "emergency" during the exposure. Over time, we also added other more calming *asanas*.

INCORPORATING TRAUMA-SENSITIVE YOGA INTO THE THERAPY PROCESS

This case clearly shows that yoga *asanas* and *pranayama* exercises cannot just simply be used for the exposure of somatic triggers. Instead, some clients initially require stable resources.

However, if there is a certain ability of affect regulation at the beginning of the therapy and clients are open to making changes— for example, mindfully feeling their feet, shoulders, etc. by moving their feet across the floor or circling their shoulders and observing the changes afterward—the yoga exercises can be virtually used as exposure to somatic triggers and woven into the therapy process. In this case, the body-oriented process-supporting work, as well as the psychoeducation and conversation on the successes or failures in mastering the triggers in everyday life, take up the largest part of the first eight to ten therapy sessions.

In the first hours, I make sure that the resources are worked out and try to avoid triggers and/or help clients to counteract them as quickly as possible with a self-calming exercise. With an increasing affect tolerance, I suggest conscious poses or breathing exercises that trigger more stress so that the clients learn to have increased tolerance for it. In this way, an exposure of somatic triggers occurs in addition to the affect regulation training. This means that avoidance is not supported. How long this phase takes and/or how quickly we can move forward depends, in turn, on the clients.

In my experience, the fear of verbalizing what happened to them decreases after about ten sessions. This can be followed by an exposure therapy in the classical sense, in which the somatic—as well as the cognitive and emotional—processing can take place. This approach can also be illustrated with a practical example (see below).

CASE EXAMPLE: MALE CLIENT

A client in his mid-thirties consulted me about his growing sleep and concentration problems. In the anamnesis, it became clear that he had suffered from physical violence, sexual violence, and neglect as a child. But he had suppressed this up to now.

Even in the first session we began with mindfulness and movement exercises—Mountain Pose, Cat–Cow, Seated Spinal Twist, and backbends—that helped him to calm himself again in moments of intense arousal. In the following four sessions, we worked out additional resources such as feeling the breath movement and calming breathing exercises such as the Bee Breath and Sun Breath. In these sessions, I consciously avoided keeping him in stress-triggering positions for too long. Instead, I suggested replacing them with resourceful poses and/or movements. I also advised him to move back and forth, which he was able to do on his own over time.

His affect tolerance became stronger and I "dared" suggest to him that he change from a resourceful pose to a stress-triggering position. I also encouraged him to observe the sensations and decide when he wanted to end this and choose something calming instead. He increasingly succeeded in mastering his emotions and sensations so that we took stock after nine sessions and then devoted ourselves to trauma memories with an exposure therapy—NET in this case.

Here is a summary of the three possibilities for planning the therapy:

- Since working out the resources cannot be done as specifically in a TSY group as in individual therapy, I recommend a course for the length of the exposure phase. Depending on the severity of the trauma, this can be between 15 and 25 group sessions.

- If we offer yoga as an element of the individual therapy, it can be good to combine the yoga elements, either before or after the therapy.

- Yoga can also be considered meaningful as process-supporting somatic exposure in the first eight to ten sessions.

12

GUIDANCE FOR INSTRUCTORS

Guiding physical exercises in the therapy is something completely different from being in a therapeutic dialog with the client. If we want to support clients in staying with themselves and being able to have personal interoceptive experiences, we must deal with such topics as voice, speaking rate, pauses, etc.

TONE OF VOICE

Trauma clients need courage if they want to face their body and physical sensations. They are probably just as afraid of sensing nothing where they should feel something as they are of feeling too much. The idea of working in a body-oriented way will presumably cause them to be stressed. A calm pitch of the voice, a soothing and encouraging way of speaking, and a relaxed, friendly face—these components are known to be activating for the ventral vagus nerve, but signal to people that they are safe.

When we guide clients, we switch to a "yoga voice," and speak somewhat more quietly, calmly, and gently, although this is not a hypnotic, monotone sing-song voice that has a sleep-inducing effect and seems to be uninvolved in what is happening. The instructions are "friendly and open," but simultaneously "clear and understandable." If clients do not know what they should do, unnecessary tension can easily arise. Get feedback about your "yoga voice" and its volume from family members or an intervision group, as well as by recording your voice to check it. Get to know various teachers, instruction styles, and voices by attending yoga courses. The voice becomes an anchor for the clients. It shows that we are entering the third space, in which we practice together.

PACE AND TIMING OF SPEECH

Interoceptive perception has its own deliberate speed and requires time, because our non-myelinated nerve fibers are slow conductors. This means that we should attune our speaking rate to allow clients adequate time to get into, sense, and release a position, or to do a breathing exercise and not feel rushed or left alone.

If we suggest an *asana* and propose staying in it for a moment, we leave clients enough time but also not too much—so this is a balancing act. If we move too quickly from one exercise to the next, the chance that clients can feel anything at all is very remote. But if we stay in a static pose with clients for too long, this can frighten them since it reminds them of being in a state of immobility. In the practice, this means that we spend a bit less time in one position with our clients when we first start practicing with them and just slowly extend the time of silent exploration. By allowing clients to decide how long they stay in one position or want to do a breathing exercise, we adapt the rhythm of instruction to their own. Although we speak at the beginning and end, clients are free at any time to decide whether they even want to get into the position and want to follow our suggestion to release it. Since we also emphasize that a pose can be released at any time or a breathing exercise can be stopped, the clients determine the pace.

PROCESSING OF INSTRUCTIONS

The instructions for yoga *asanas* are often quite complex, and there is a tendency to give too many of them at once. When this involves interceptive perception, people are not capable of processing multiple types of information at one time. We are therefore initially satisfied with a few fundamental statements when guiding an exercise, and can gradually include additional elements later. When first practicing Tree Pose—in which we stand on one foot and place the second foot on the ankle of the first—we direct attention to the supporting leg, for example. Practitioners can then initially observe its musculature and the little balancing movements. In a later phase, we invite our clients to pay attention to the position of the pelvis and lower back. If they tend to have a sway back, we correct this verbally. In a further step, we may suggest paying attention to the muscles of shoulder area. Everything at once would be overwhelming and thwart our therapeutic goals.

When treating trauma clients, I recommend proceeding cautiously and initially keeping the focus on external details. For example: "In this pose, the right arm points in the direction of the window and the left arm toward the opposite wall." It helps beginners to look at the surroundings: Where is the window? Where is the wall? Where are my arms in this space? If they still have very little body awareness, this outer focus can initially "replace" sensing. In addition, this approach provides orientation in the here and now, in space, and in the present. It helps clients to feel a stronger sense of safety.

Instructions for the perception of an inner focus could be given with following comments, for example: "You may sense the tension in your shoulder muscles or even the stretch of your arms. You may also notice how your ribs move when you breathe, for example."

People can process more instructions and do so more quickly with an external focus than with inner attention. More time is required for developing the inner attention, and it is not possible to focus on as many details. You can test this yourself: Stretch your right arm and hand horizontally at shoulder height, then look to see whether your arm and hand are in the desired position. You can see the result with one glance. Let your arm come back down. Now close your eyes and follow these same instructions one more time. It takes more time to feel the exact location of your arm and hand.

STAYING IN CONTACT

We stay in verbal contact with clients through our voice. Relationship traumas in particular are so disturbing because the caregiver has broken off contact and not restored it. In many cases, the perpetrator acted in complete silence or had only given the affected person attention during the abuse, breaking off contact afterward. It is also not uncommon for children to have experienced weeks of silence as a punishment from their parents or carers.

When the contact is broken off, this leads to a feeling of being completely lost. In the beginning, we do not have any long breaks in speaking. If we do, we announce them ahead of time. Interruptions in the flow of speech that are too long can unsettle clients, who are very much in danger of dissociating in this case. We support clients by describing the movement process and its variations regarding how they enter into an *asana*, as well as by remaining audible while we hold an *asana*. Our suggestions for interoceptive sensations and variation possibilities while holding the *asana*, as well as releasing it and noticing sensations, help clients to orient themselves in the here and now.

KEEPING THE FOCUS ON THE BODY

If we want to help clients regain and expand their interoceptive abilities, it is absolutely necessary to orient our way of speaking toward this goal. Verbal instructions should therefore not distract their attention to things outside of the body such as sounds or objects in the room. We should likewise avoid evoking visualizations and inner images. We can mention very concrete and functional muscles, breath movements, joints, bones, etc. since this way of experiencing the body and one's own corporeality does not usually have negative connotations. Then it becomes easier for the affected person to deal with their own body. Through its function, the body becomes experienceable, comprehensible, and tangible. Since we all share the experience of the human body, our own sensations are teachers that whisper the ideas to us. Just imagining what could happen is not enough.

The following example is for a standing forward bend:

> When you are ready, you can go into a forward bend. You decide how deep you would like to go… And while you do this, you can perhaps notice in which of your muscles you sense a stretch…this may be on the back of your legs…or in your back…you may even notice the weight of your upper body or arms…

This is where the therapeutic dialog starts. We share what we feel with each other. This can lead to surprising insights. For example, I occasionally miss some sensations and clients draw my attention to them. Such moments promote the relationship. I do not create them intentionally since they simply happen due to this type of setting. Interoceptive yoga is a work-in.

Avoid questions such as:

- "What are you feeling?"

- "Do you sense a difference?"

- "Are you feeling the floor beneath your feet?"

- "Can you notice the tension in your leg muscles?"

Questions like these can turn yoga exercises into a task that feels like an obligation. If clients do not succeed in following the instructions, their thoughts are stimulated and emotions triggered:

- *Failure:* "I should be able to feel this."

- *Helplessness:* "I don't know how I should do this."

- *Despair:* "I still can't feel this."

- *Anger:* "I hate that I constantly have to deal with this damn body."

Clients who are no longer connected with their body and the felt sense try to cope with the stress that has been triggered. In addition, such questions direct the clients' attention to the outside and to us since they imply that they must answer them and/or justify themselves.

We select phrases that allow clients to remain with themselves:

- "Perhaps you sense the stretch at the back of your thigh muscles…"

- "Sometimes the difference between right and left can be sensed immediately, and it occasionally can only be recognized later."

- "When you activate your muscles, you may notice that they start to tremble after a while."

- "When you balance yourself, you may feel the activity of the muscles in the standing leg and possibly some little movements to balance yourself."

- "After we have released the pose, a difference between right and left can sometimes be felt."

- "Perhaps you can notice how your breath gradually calms down."

- "It's interesting to observe the movement in your elbow joint as you do this."

- "It's possible that you feel nothing at all, and that is also completely okay" (cf. also Emerson and Hopper 2011).

When we have practiced an *asana* over a longer time, I make less specific statements than at the start. This can be illustrated with the example of the side bend, which is more specific in the beginning:

> We are going into a side bend to the right... You may feel how your intercostal muscles are extending...and possibly also notice a difference between your ribs on the right and those on the left side or in your chest... What you may also feel is the weight of your right arm that hangs down... If you feel nothing like this at all, this shouldn't disturb you.

Later, the statement is less specific:

> We are going into a side bend to the right...and I invite you to notice what happens in your muscles...where they are stretched and which ones are active... You may also notice differences between right and left...possibly in your chest...or in your arms.

EMPHASIS ON CHOICES AND FREEDOM IN DECISION-MAKING

In most studies that are concerned with the effect of yoga, there is no allusion to the idea that the type of instruction must be adapted in any way to the needs of trauma clients. One exception is the work of Emerson and his team. They emphasize how important it is that our instructions—quite to the contrary of classic yoga—are formulated in an inviting way and should imply choices (cf. also Emerson and Hopper 2011).

Clear instructions provide structure and support, and therefore a sense of safety, and this is something that clients urgently need at the beginning of the therapy. If we open up a space in which "everything is possible," we overwhelm clients. In the confrontation with a new experience, most people quickly become aware of whether they want to get involved or not—and they act correspondingly. The situation is different for people suffering from complex trauma. The lack of defensive strategies leads them to habitual dissociation as soon as they feel overwhelmed. They generally cannot actively escape since they often lack points of reference. They have very little body awareness and therefore hardly any somatic markers to make this decision possible for them. Such clients benefit from structure and a sense of safety.

On the other hand, we are interested in offering a setting in the therapy that differs to the maximum degree from the trauma experience of not having any choice and being helplessly at the mercy of one's own emotions. We would like to give clients adequate control—transparency is what allows people to experience a sense of security and the feeling of not being at anyone's mercy. This is why we explore our concrete ideas and make suggestions for our approach, as well as the next steps, with the clients in psychoeducation.

This type of clarification is an essential component of working with people who suffer from complex trauma. We do it intensively at the start of the therapy, but it remains an important element throughout its entire course. Second, a sense of security arises when individuals know that they are free at any time to decide against something without having to fear negative consequences. These premises apply to both the "classic" therapeutic interventions and those that are related to the body.

In relation to bodywork in trauma therapy, we primarily provide structure and security at the start. As soon as clients become familiar with body-related interventions, more space for making choices gradually develops. A female client had this to say about it:

> At the start, when we first began the session with yoga, I was happy that you told me what I should do. I could hold onto that and follow your instructions. At that point in time, I wasn't able to decide about things. That would have frightened me. It took some time for me to open up a little to it, notice sensations, and draw my conclusions—which means making my own choice. At the start of the therapy, I felt almost nothing. How should I have known whether I should do it one way or the other?

So we must find a balance between structure and the freedom to make decisions. When we are in contact with our clients, we get feedback on how much structure and freedom they need and/or "tolerate." If they have too little body awareness at the start of the bodywork, a clear structure helps the clients to basically open up to it. Too many variations are often perceived as overwhelming during this phase. If they are even done at all, they are performed rather mechanically. My instructions are friendly, open, and formulated "softly," but just as clear and distinct. I am restrained with my offer of variations. Only with time, when they have developed more contact with their own body, can clients use this feedback and make decisions. Then they can also truly benefit from having choices.

EXAMPLE FOR OFFERING CHOICE

At the beginning of the bodywork, we set up an *asana* together, such as Warrior Pose. My formulations sound like this:

> I would like to invite you to try a powerful *asana*, Warrior I. To do this, we first stand up straight…and move the right foot a big step to the front. The left leg stays stretched toward the back while we bend the right leg a little.

> …Activate your stomach muscles so that your lumbar spine is protected. Now you can try out something like pressing the heel of your left leg into the floor…and releasing it again… And perhaps you can sense the stretch of the back leg muscles.

So my instructions are very concrete and comprehensible.

If we have made progress in the practice, variations can help the clients in making decisions. Based on the above example, this can look like this:

> I suggest that you try a powerful pose, Warrior I. To do this, we first stand up straight… Now we move the right foot a big step to the front and activate the stomach muscles… At this point, you may want to pause for a moment and get a sense of how large you would like to make this step…somewhat bigger…or smaller… Or does it feel just right to you?

> …Take your time… When you feel what is happening in the back leg, you can press your heel into the floor, for example… And you may feel the stretch of the back leg muscles… You can also experiment with taking some of the pressure off this back leg by slightly bending your knee… What feels right to you at this moment?

We should also be clear about serving as the model and standard on which the clients orient themselves. The way in which we instruct and show the *asana* is how it should be. For some clients, this already excludes a freedom of choice. As an example of this, here are the instructions for a side bend: "We go into a slight side bend and extend our right side. 'Slight' can mean like this for you… [I bend just a little]…or like this [I bend a bit more, but not to the maximum extent]. There are no right or wrong side bends." By being open to the clients and mirroring their variations of the positions, we do not awaken their false ambitions of having to do it like we do.

It is not advisable to praise clients because they use the alternatives that we offer. The old pattern of wanting to please can have the effect that they dutifully do what is expected of them and apparently make a decision but are not at all centered within themselves and their experience.

Here are some formulations for choices (cf. also Emerson and Hopper 2011):

- "If you like…"

- "If it feels appropriate for you…"

- "Perhaps…"

- "You can try…"

- "I invite you to…"

- "You can adapt the suggestions at any time and change them…"

- "End the position as soon as you feel uneasy or something similar…"

- "You decide how long you want to hold this *asana* today."

- "Notice how it feels to you today."

- "Try it out to see how high you would like to take your arms today."

- "You decide how it is appropriate for you."

- "You can end the pose at any time."

- "You determine the intensity and length of time."

CORRECTIONS

As already mentioned, we basically demonstrate the *asanas*, practice them with the clients, and only correct verbally—not hands on. Although this is not a problem for most yoga positions, we should have enough experience and body awareness to avoid demonstrating errors that the clients could copy. We should also be clear about where there could be a risk of injury and what we should pay attention to when giving instructions, as well as in which cases we should end an *asana*. Care should be taken with the knees, lumbar spine, and cervical spine:

Knees: The bent knee, such as in Warrior I and II, should be placed behind or vertically above the ankle and not in front of it when exerting pressure. At the same time, be sure that the knee joint does not rotate to the right or left side (see Chapter 13).

Lumbar vertebrae: The natural rotation is just 3–5 degrees. To avoid a more intense rotation in positions like Spinal Twist, the stomach muscles should be activated to achieve stabilization in this area.

Lack of tension in the stomach muscles during various *asanas* such as Tree Pose can lead to a sway back and result in backaches.

Cervical vertebrae: When tilting the upper body backward, we must pay attention that the head is not placed too far in the nape of the neck or even "dropped." Instead, controlled and gentle movements should be used.

We consciously address these vulnerable areas and use a concrete example to demonstrate what we mean. If our verbal corrections are not accepted because the clients do not understand them, we gently direct them out of the *asana* or turn it into an interoceptive awareness exercise. For example, if clients place their knees in front of the ankle instead of vertically in Warrior Pose:

> Maybe you can take a look at your knee and see where it is right now. When we spend more time in a position that is strenuous for the knee joint—like the Warrior—it is better to have it behind the ankle or vertically above it.

We demonstrate this and show the various positions so that our clients can get a clear idea of it:

> So you can try this out to see how it is to move the knee back, perhaps even quite a bit behind the ankle…and then right above it again… You may feel a difference or perhaps you won't. It helps me to take another look if I'm not sure about it.

This is a good opportunity to present the "message" of self-care without explicitly addressing it.

Many yoga books discuss "mistakes" that must be corrected such as pulled-up shoulders, locked knees, or a sunken chest. When working with clients, errors are not commented on or corrected, so that the clients do not feel like failures. These habitual postures are often related to trauma and can only be changed gradually. We can turn the frozen poses or movements into an interoceptive exercise by exploring the sensations of the pulled-up shoulders together with the clients, for example. Another example is exploring the difference between a sunken chest and a wide, open posture together with the clients. Over the course of time, clients become aware of their posture tendencies and start to change them. They often notice that they assume an accustomed posture and address it on their own. We can invite them to explore this programming and experiment with changes so that they can always make the decision as to the extent to which they can tolerate postural changes. The *asanas* are bridges that help people to train awareness and to sense themselves.

THE LANGUAGE OF EMPOWERMENT

The choice of words and expressions is very important in trauma therapy, and the same principle applies to bodywork. Whatever we say has much weight. We consciously choose a language of empowerment that leads clients to experiences of security and control. For example, I use expressions such as "choose," "determine," "as you see fit," "…up to you," "decide," etc., to make clients aware that they are not at my mercy and can very well influence their own mental states. Words like "choose" or "decide" are often either empty phrases or triggers at the beginning. This changes over the course of time since purely cognitive concepts can become lived body experiences through the practical exercises. I like to use the word "empowerment."

To get a clear sense of the effects created by something like changing a posture, I generally use a scale from 0–10, which corresponds with the SUD Scale (Subjective Units of Distress): 0 is a relaxed state in which clients feel good, safe, and calm, while 10 embodies the worst possible degree of stress, fear, etc. I ask about this scale on a regular basis at the start of the therapy. Once clients achieve a decrease on the stress curve when they practice, I consciously draw their attention to it: "By deciding to do xyz, your fear was reduced from 8 to 5." This intervention reminds clients time and again that they are able to influence things.

WAVELIKE INSTRUCTION AND BREAKS

In order to experience an *asana*, it is important to observe the phases of entering into it, holding it, releasing it, and noticing sensations afterward. The phase of noticing sensations supports inner collection and is especially important for trauma clients. This is where they can have the experience that activation is—automatically, and without any personal actions—followed by calming. The observation of this process, whether during the breath, heartbeat, or in the musculature, strengthens the client's trust in their own body. The "wavelike" structuring of a yoga sequence—which means breaks for noticing sensations, as well as the calming *asanas*—teaches clients to deal with the "gas pedal" and the "brake." At this point I would like to mention once again that even Warrior Pose can have a calming effect. We should not make the error of already knowing what will have a calming and what will have an activating effect.

In alternating between tension and/or effort and the subsequent recuperation, the body- and movement-oriented work opens up and increases access to the elastic 30 to 70 percent activation in which we normally move during everyday life. This is because clients gradually learn to tolerate and control their body sensations and affects.

If we encourage clients to follow how a tension dissolves, a stretch decreases, and exertion becomes relaxation, they will not only gain stronger trust in the change itself; they learn that things can take a turn for the better. By pointing out this phenomenon to clients over and over again, they will gradually become more conscious of it.

Clients benefit greatly from this idea in everyday life. Up to now they may have only noticed the worsening of their mental states. According to one client, "Today I also register the nuances. For example, I noticed that I wasn't feeling well in the morning but this improved somewhat in the afternoon. Noticing this causes joy and trust that things could get even better."

RELATIONSHIPS AND MIRRORING

Successful relationships are very much based on how the "intercorporeality" was and is experienced. Maurice Merleau-Ponty described this in his book, *The World of Perception* (2004). It means that we first experience our counterpart through their physical expression. Even before we reflect the person across from us, their expression makes a physical impression on us. Seen from this perspective, the basis for the social exchange is intercorporeal resonance (Fuchs 2008).

When this phenomenon is scientifically researched, we find ourselves in the field of social synchrony—the observed physical synchronization within a social interaction system that usually occurs spontaneously without being planned and/or perceived by the involved person. We already find early imitation in newborns (Meltzoff and Moore 1983). This is where statements about attachment styles can be made (Isabella and Belsky 1991). Mutual chronologically coordinated interaction behavior, which means synchronous interaction, can primarily be observed in secure attachment styles. Synchrony also correlates with the sympathy of the involved person and therefore with the quality of the relationship. When these findings are associated with the therapy relationship, it has been possible to prove in studies that primarily unapproachable, introverted, and insecure people have a negative correlation with synchrony.

So if we take into account attachment experiences in our considerations, it becomes clear that insecurely attached children grow into adults who have difficulty with interpersonal contact. They have not experienced this natural mirroring, and are also unable to learn it to an adequate degree. These circumstances are often encountered in the therapy setting by applying the "technique" of mirroring. However, if we, as therapists, do not enter into an honest resonance with clients, this approach can easily fail and even cause the opposite of the desired effect. In the body therapy setting, we attempt to respond to this danger by always participating. This quite naturally results in the experience of synchronicity.

In practice, we constantly alternate roles in mirroring and leading. We give instructions and the clients assume our posture. We suggest variations and the clients try them out. They decide on a variation. Then we mirror the clients by assuming their posture. We initially also mirror the "errors" such as pulled-up shoulders, tensed legs, etc., because this gives us a better feeling for the physical sensations of our counterparts. Time and again, we attempt to transition into leading by letting our shoulders drop down and observing whether our clients automatically follow. If they do so, we can ask them to perceive how their shoulders or their breath, etc., now feel. Or we can assume the leadership by—as already mentioned above—suggesting an exercise in which the shoulders are consciously pulled up and lowered again, for example.

People who do not feel good in their body become insecure when they are observed. As a result, we never sit directly across from the clients but always choose an offset position. This is another way that we contribute to clients not feeling observed.

In TSY there is no right or wrong. All that exists is the personal experience, which is always appreciated. We do not touch the clients. We do not tell them how an *asana* should feel or which effect it should have. Only the interoceptive experiences count. We do not know whether a position done in a different way will feel "better." With our suggestions, we solely open up the space for exploring something new. Instead, we say: "If this position feels unpleasant to you, you can modify it and discover how that feels." We show a variation, but do not have any expectation of the result. Our offer of a relationship is based on an equal footing. The clients do not need to interact and be in a relationship with us, react, or justify themselves—which may sometimes overwhelm them. We stand side by side and enter the transitional space together.

INTEROCEPTIVE LANGUAGE

In TSY we speak concretely about interoceptive sensations such as temperature, weight, stretching, relaxation, balance, etc., and direct the focus time and again to physical sensations. We use a structural language and name the joints, muscles, and bones (cf. Emerson and Hopper 2011; Ogden *et al.* 2006). Our personal observations in a position or during a breath exercise give us points of reference.

Interoceptive sensations may be:

- weight on muscles and bones

- weight of a body part

- tensing of a muscle

- relaxation of a muscle

- movement

- pressure through contact with the chair/floor or on a part of the body (hand on thigh)

- diminishing of pressure—relief

- temperature in the body or surroundings and temperature differences

- temperature of a contact surface

- texture

- equilibrium and balance

- stretch and pull

- expansiveness

- tension, activity, strength, and trembling

- relaxation and heaviness

- pulse and heartbeat

- movement of the breath.

As already explained in the above examples, we consciously address the interoceptive possibilities and make clients aware of possible somatosensory experiences.

PART V

PRACTICE

The heart of this book is concerned with yoga *asanas*, *pranayama*, and mindfulness in practice. We learn yoga as mindfulness in movement and breath in three steps. We first embrace our own presence and awareness in the body during breathing and practicing. Our mental focus is on our physical sensations. In the next step, our attention turns to our thoughts, emotions, and sensations. Observing and mastering them creates a feeling of strength and empowerment. The last step—the actual meditation in motion—leads to a relaxed body that perceives its intuitive impulses and can follow them (cf. Faulds 2005).

As already mentioned, therapists are not the experts in Trauma-Sensitive Yoga (TSY). Both therapist and client are students who gather experiences and explore their own interoception. This allows them to examine the effect and efficacy of the measures, as well as to grasp and constantly improve their personal affect regulation. As trauma therapists, this means that we are willing to face our own somatosensory experiences and the challenges that we encounter in all three of these steps.

In the practice section you will find exercises that are marked with an asterisk. They are initially meant to serve the improvement of our own interoception and to give us a feeling for our own body and body awareness. So let's get started with the poses and movements.

13

ASANAS

On the one hand, the *asanas* in yoga are static postures that are assumed with mindfulness, held, and released in turn. They are connected into a type of choreography. On the other hand, *asanas* can be performed as dynamic movements: gently, slowly, powerfully, quickly, rhythmically, or synchronized with the breath. In addition, *asanas* can help us to train mindful observation of interoceptive experiences, as well as emotional and mental waves.

Here are a few brief exercises to provide an understanding of the various possibilities offered by interoceptive perception.

EXERCISE: BALANCE

The balance system perceives every change in our position in space.

Stand upright. If you are not accustomed to balance exercises, do this close to a wall so that you can lean against it if necessary. Now shift your weight to your right leg, and then place your left foot on your right ankle. For a better sense of balance, fix your eyes on a fixed point that is one to two yards away. Your arms can either hang relaxed at your side or be bent with your hands folded in front of your heart.

What do you observe in your body? Which muscles are working to keep you in balance? How has your breath changed? How are you compensating for swaying? For a bit more of a challenge, close your eyes for a brief moment. What do you observe now?

*EXERCISE: AWARENESS OF THERMORECEPTORS

Thermoreceptors measure the heat, cold, and temperature differences. Strenuous poses can produce heat, so changing your place can allow you to feel the coolness on the floor.

Consciously inhale through your nose with your mouth closed and you will notice the cooling air on your nasal walls. Feel the temperature difference of the air that you exhale. Explore this by inhaling through your mouth and noticing the temperature difference between the inhale and the exhale.

*EXERCISE: BECOMING FAMILIAR WITH ENTEROCEPTION

Enteroceptors are responsible for the perception of organ activity. For example, they measure the pulse and heartbeat.

Stand upright and notice your pulse and breath frequency. Now do ten squats and notice the change of your heartbeat and breath frequency. Pay attention to whether you notice any other changes. Stay in a state of mindful observation until your pulse and breath frequency have normalized again. What do you feel when you direct your attention to calming yourself?

What follows are examples of *asanas* I use in TSY. They can all be done in everyday clothing and don't require any preparation. They can be done on a chair and standing (cf. also Adkins, Robinson, and Stewart 2011; Emerson and Hopper 2011; Rohnfeld 2011).

The classification of the *asanas* into basic poses, as well as calming and stimulating exercises, should be understood as guidelines that do not apply to everyone. A forward bend can be calming for some clients but produce an activating or frightening effect for others. Every *asana* and breathing exercise must be carefully introduced and examined for its individual effect together with the clients. It is therefore counterproductive if we label exercises such as in the following: "This is a calming *asana.*" If our clients have a completely different experience, this can trigger their feeling of having failed. They may become insecure and mistrust therapists in the future. Remember that we are only interested in exploring and observing. By labeling an exercise, we violate this principle and restrict ourselves and our clients. In any case, we must still check to see whether this exercise actually has a calming effect, in which way, etc.

I recommend that therapists first try out every *asana* to explore the respective effects on our own person. Although it is obvious that our sensations will be different from those of our clients, we all share the experiences of a human body, and this at the least allows some conclusions about how another person could feel in a certain posture. The classification in the following section is meant only for therapists as a better overview; it is not generally valid.

Each *asana* has its own instructional text. These instructions contain many aspects that are intended as suggestions. However, we should never suggest more than one or two possibilities at a time.

The examples of instructions and formulation are presented in the form of a "monolog," but in the one-to-one setting we are in contact with our clients and mutually explore which effect a posture has. For examples of how such dialogs can be designed, see Chapter 12.

When I teach TSY in a group, I hold a "monolog" in which I offer variations and choices. Then I leave it up to each individual to make use of them (cf. Emerson and Hopper 2011) and to have their own experiences.

I usually start with setting up the basic posture—seated or standing Mountain Pose. These are good choices since they are the starting point for many variations, allow choices, and make it easy to return to this position time and again when practicing them. This gives them the character of being familiar and trusted, communicating a sense of security and grounding to the clients. Instructions (and photos) for these poses are given in this chapter.

Basic seated poses: Centering and arriving

- Mountain Pose
- Seated Spinal Twist

Arriving in Mountain Pose and Seated Spinal Twist can also have a calming effect.

Seated *asanas* for calming: Activating the parasympathetic nervous system

- Forward bend
- Torso circles
- Cat–Cow Pose
- Variations of Cat–Cow Pose
- Gentle side bend

Seated *asanas* for activation: Activating the sympathetic nervous system

- Backbend
- Dynamic side bend
- Staff Pose
- Chair Position
- Boat Pose
- Triangle Pose

Basic standing poses: Centering and arriving

- Mountain Pose
- Tree Pose

Asanas for calming (without illustrations): Activating the parasympathetic nervous system

- Gentle side bend right and left (cf. seated side bend)
- Gentle balance exercises—shifting weight to the right/left, front/back
- Forward bend (cf. seated side bend)

Activating poses: Activating the sympathetic nervous system

- Warrior I Pose
- Warrior II Pose
- Downward Dog Pose and Three-Legged Dog Pose with chair
- Downward Dog Pose and Three-Legged Dog Pose without chair

Every static pose allows us to explore immobility and silence, as well as the movement of the breath since it moves the body in a variety of ways. Every static posture can transition into a dynamic movement that can sometimes be synchronized with the breath movements virtually on its own. In a forward bend, this can be a slight to and fro movement. In the Warrior Poses this can be a gentle or dynamic up and down movement, etc. As already mentioned, silence and being static can awaken memories of feeling helpless and immobility. So a reminder about the movement of the breath is important since some clients tend to hold it as they fixate on their lack of motion when they are in a stiff posture.

The flow of the breath is a main element of classic yoga. In TSY, it has a special value since the held breath signals danger to the body and can become a trigger. If we occasionally observe our own flow of breath, we will catch ourselves holding it time and again. This is a good time to remind clients of their breath. Being able to breathe freely during exertion communicates this message to the body: "I am safe here." I explain this to clients until they are capable of remembering their breathing, as well as becoming aware of the breath's significance and their possibilities for controlling it (see also Chapter 14).

SOME PRELIMINARY REMARKS
ABOUT THE INSTRUCTIONS

- Each *asana* has an instruction text that contains many interoceptive suggestions. Always just use one or at most two suggestions and allow clients enough time to follow these ideas.

- Before each exercise, directly address the affected body parts and muscles by emphasizing to the clients that this involves their body. Instead of saying "the knee or the calves" in your instructions, always use "your knees or your calves."

- Don't ask questions such as: "Do you feel the muscles in your upper arms?" This can really distress clients if they do not feel these muscles.

- It's fine to repeat phrases. Just as in the exercises, a sense of security is more important than the range of variation and diversity.

- The three dots (…) mean that you give clients enough time at this point to assume a pose and/or notice the body sensations. You can bridge longer pauses by making comments on what you are doing and/or what you see. For example, if you have suggested exploring the sit bones through little movements on the chair and the clients have begun doing so, you can comment on this in the following way: "…just like that, little movements to the right and left." Sometimes even just an "exactly" is enough to shorten a pause and give clients the feeling that you are there and that they are doing it right.

ADDITIONAL COMMENTS

Many of the *asanas* were developed from Mountain Pose. There are instructions for seated variations and the standing variations below.

I recommend having blankets or cushions available, so that clients can adapt their seat heights, for example.

SEATED POSES
SEATED CENTERING POSES
MOUNTAIN POSE

Seated starting position; firmness and calm; neutral position that we can always return to.

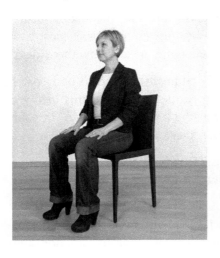 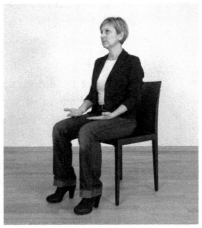

I would like to invite you to join me in getting into Mountain Pose, a basic posture in yoga. It's best to first make yourself comfortable on the chair... For all of the *asanas*, you can keep your eyes open or closed and change this at any time... When you are ready, place your feet at hip width on the floor. You can also try out how it feels if you place them closer together or further apart...

Perhaps you would first like to make contact with your feet... There are various possibilities to do this. You can move your feet back and forth... You can bend and stretch your toes...feel the texture of the floor...and you may also take a look at your feet. Perhaps you feel your feet and perhaps the contact with the ground... You may not even feel anything at all and this is completely okay.

If you let your attention wander further up, you will come to your calves...and your knees. In case you notice that the chair is too high or too low, you can use a pillow or blanket to correct it. Take a moment... and let your attention keep wandering upward to your knees... When you let your perception move to the points and areas where your body touches the chair, you may feel your sit bones... In order to reassure yourself and intensify this feeling, simply rock to and fro a little...or move back and forth.

As soon as it feels appropriate to you, direct your attention to your spinal column and lengthen it a little in the direction of the ceiling. Take your time.

VARIATIONS OF MOUNTAIN POSE

You can sit up straight in the chair...and then sink back down into it a bit... You decide how big the movement should be...and repeat this several times to explore your personal form of straightening up... When you turn your attention to your shoulders, you may now notice tension... And if it feels appropriate to you, you can move your shoulders a little bit...however this feels appropriate to you right now. If you like, you can do circles...or pull them up and let them slide back down again... But you can also keep your shoulders stable and still... Another possibility is massaging your shoulders a bit with your hands.

Your hands can rest on your thighs or you can place them with the palms up...and you may notice a difference in how your hands and arms feel in the respective positions...you may sense the material under your hands. Perhaps you feel this even more clearly when you move your hands... Try it out... You may even notice a difference in relation to the texture of the material or your body temperature through it. If you like, you can focus your attention on the *movements* caused by your breath. I invite you to observe this rhythm... Perhaps you notice it more in your chest or more in your belly... Maybe you notice that the movements are distinct or very gentle. You don't have to follow a concept and try to breathe in a certain way.

MOVEMENT POSSIBILITIES IN MOUNTAIN POSE

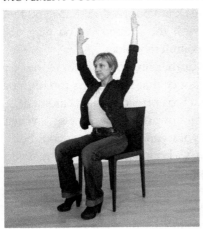 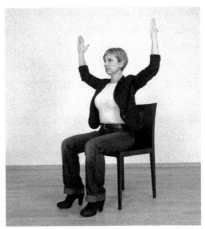

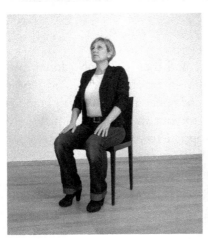 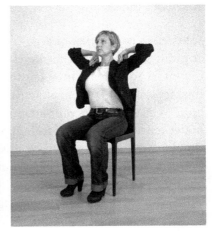

- Stretch and bend your arms.
- Pull up your shoulders and let them come down again.

- Move your arms up and down at your sides or in front of your body.

- Circle your arms.

- Tilt your head to the right and to the left or circle it—these are little movements.

- Raise your head slightly (don't overextend your cervical spine), and then tilt it slightly to the back, in alternation.

- Turn your head to the right and then the left.

- Tilt your head to the right and then the left side.

SPINAL TWIST
Stability in the center; opening and stretching the chest muscles; change of perspective.

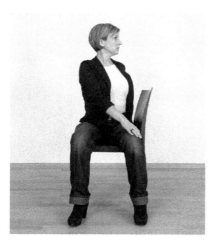

(We start in Mountain Pose.) I would like to invite you to do an *asana* in which we move the thoracic vertebrae and change our perspective. To protect your spinal column, it's good to first sit taller... To stabilize your lumbar spine, pull in your navel toward your spinal column... This allows your lower back to remain stable while you turn your upper body. To get familiar with this feeling of the stable center, try out how it feels to pull in your navel and then let it go again... Perhaps you feel your abdominal muscles... If you like, put one hand on your belly...and you may notice a movement beneath your hand...through this tensing and relaxing... Sometimes it is helpful to take a look at your hand to see the movement...

When you are ready, place your right hand on your left thigh... activate your navel point...and turn your upper body to the left... your left arm can hang down in a relaxed way...or you can just as well stretch it to the back...and intensify the stretch as a result... Try out whatever is appropriate for you at this moment... You can look over your left shoulder...or also to the side... You are always in control of how far you would like to turn... The twist may make you aware of the muscles between your shoulder blades...and you may notice how your ribs move when you breathe. Perhaps you notice the weight of your left arm...or a stretch in your throat and neck...or the difference between the right and left shoulder...

You can stay here a little bit longer...perhaps for three to four breaths...or come back into a neutral posture at your own speed. Give your body time to relax and notice any possible changes in the muscles or breathe as you do so. Then turn to the other side.

CALMING SEATED POSES
FORWARD BEND
Stretching the back muscles; feeling the weight of the upper body and the head.

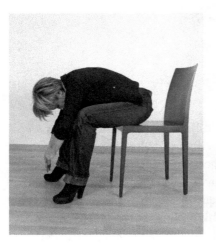 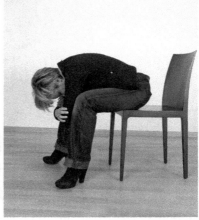

This posture lengthens the back and stretches the back muscles. To do the forward bend, it is helpful to place the feet a bit wider apart so that the upper body has space... Take a moment to find the appropriate position for your feet...and then bend your upper body forward at your own tempo... You decide how you want to hold your hands and arms: either cross your arms by holding your elbows...or simply let your arms hang down... Try out both possibilities, and then decide which one is appropriate for you at this moment... While your breath continues to flow, I would like to invite you to focus on your back and neck muscles. Perhaps you feel a stretch... Or you mainly feel the sensation of weight in your arms or your head... Perhaps you don't sense anything at all...or something entirely different... This is completely okay... If you feel like it, you can move your head with a nod, or left and right like a "no." You decide how long you would like to stay in the forward bend...and can end this posture at any time. You can return to the starting posture at your own pace... Perhaps you feel an impulse to move in another direction...or to stretch. Take the time to sense what your body is telling you.

PRACTICE TIP: If we have only practiced these *asanas* with each other a few times, I do not explicitly speak about breathing at this point since the breath and its movements are restricted in this position due to the compression of the abdomen. Focusing on this can cause fear. After a certain accustoming to this position, the breath can also be addressed with a statement like this: "You may sense the movement of your breath more to the side or also slight movements in the back. You can sit up a bit straighter at any time and see how far you would like to bend forward at this moment."

Especially in this posture, clients may feel a growing sense of empowerment when they notice that they can sit up straight and immediately change the impressions and feelings. This posture usually has a calming effect. However, it can also promote a dissociative state when clients habitually use it as a protection mechanism.

TORSO CIRCLES

Bringing movement into play; synchronizing movement with the breath; feeling a weight shift.

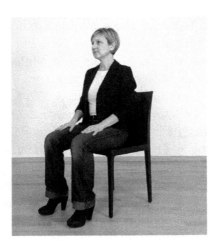

(We start in Mountain Pose.) For this *asana*, we need a bit of space in the back...so slide a little forward on the chair... Take your time to find a position that is comfortable for you...

As you let your breath flow, you can lean back a bit with a straight back... Try out how far...and activate your abdominal muscles as you do so... You can stay here for a while...and allow your breath to keep flowing... Observe where you feel your breath at the moment... Perhaps you would like to come forward again... The speed is up to you... Your back always stays straight... You can repeat this movement for several times... You decide how far you want to lean back or come to the front each time anew. You may enjoy turning this into a rhythmic movement...by moving back and forth at your own pace... and coordinating this with your breath... Inhale when you lean back and exhale when you come to the front.

... Another variation is rocking from side to side...and you may notice that this requires different muscles... If you like, you can do the side-to-side rocking motion for a few breaths...or whether you want to return to the back-and-forth movement...or...find another possibility and combine the two movements so you round the corners into a circle... You can do smaller or bigger circles. You determine the size of your circles... You can change the size at any time... If you like, you can continue circling in the same direction or...if it feels appropriate to you, you can also change the direction… Perhaps both directions feel identical or you sense a difference…or a preferred direction…

Make another four or five circling movements…and then return to the center at your own speed… You can allow the circles to get smaller and smaller or simply return to the center—whatever you prefer.

PRACTICE TIP: The gentle torso circles can also be synchronized with the breath. Inhale when the upper body moves and exhale when it comes to the front. Since the exercise requires more concentration, I only suggest it once clients are accustomed to synchronizing movement and breath.

GENTLE SIDE BEND
Feeling the stretch and weight; differentiated perceiving of differences.

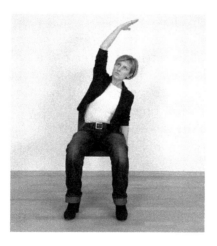

(We start in Mountain Pose.) We can now bring stretching and movement into play at any time by raising the right arm… You can allow your left arm to hang down in a relaxed way…or support it by placing your hand on your upper thigh…or find a different place for the arm that feels appropriate at the moment… You can keep your right arm stretched… or even slightly bent…whatever feels appropriate to you.

When you have found your position, bend your upper body a little to the left… Your arm follows the movement as far as you like… One variation is to pull your stretched right arm to the left and…perhaps feel a difference in the stretch of your arm muscles as you do so…

and in your right side…perhaps also feel the weight in your arm. It may occur to you that your right side has less weight on the chair… If you focus on your breathing, you may notice that it has changed… and may act differently on the right side than the left… Perhaps you discover that the tilt restricts the movement of the breath.

Stay in your pose for another three to four breaths or bring your right arm down again. How long you would like to stay in a pose is always your decision. You can end it at any time… If you give yourself a moment to notice the body sensations, you may sense differences between the right and the left… If you don't sense anything right now, this is absolutely okay. Perceiving nothing is also a perception.

Once you are ready, we will change sides. Now I invite you to lift your left arm. You determine how you would like to hold your right arm and where you want to place it or your hand… You can do this in the same way on the other side or in an entirely different way…

PRACTICE TIP: To draw the client's attention to differences in perception, we can also compare two *asanas* with each other. For example, allow them to observe the breath movement in Mountain Pose and ask how they perceive the breathing at this moment. Then go into the side bend to make a comparison. You can repeat this a few times.

You can do the same with the position of the shoulders, your weight on the chair, and many other interoceptive perceptions.

CAT–COW POSE
Bringing movement into play; synchronizing breath with movement; alternating between an activating and a calming posture.

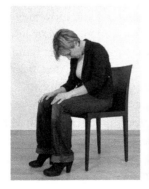 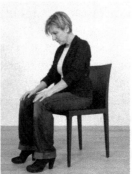 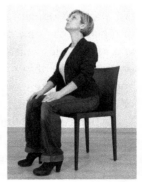

When the forward bend is combined with the backbend, a movement of the spinal column occurs that is called the *Cat–Cow* in yoga... I invite you to try this movement... We start by rounding the back...by bending your upper body... You decide how much you want to curve your spinal column as you do it... Rest your hands on your thigh... When you have arrived in the position of the Cat, start moving upward again... Straighten your spinal column at your own pace until you come into a slight backbend—the Cow... Once again, how far you want to bend backward is up to you...but be gentle with your cervical spine and don't allow your head to go back too far.

Now you can decide on your rhythm and repeat the movement several times at your own pace... If it feels appropriate to you or you are not already doing this automatically, you can synchronize this movement with your breath rhythm... Exhale when you bend forward...and inhale as soon as you come up again... You determine your rhythm and pace... You can also choose a different rhythm than the breath...

In the next step, I would like to invite you to direct your attention to the movement of your upper body... You may especially notice the movement in your back as it bends and stretches...or in your belly, which sometimes has more space and sometimes less...or in your chest... You may possibly notice completely different sensations while you move in your own rhythm... We could do three or four movements together...and when you are ready, find your way back to a neutral position...and take a moment to notice the sensations in your body...

PRACTICE TIP: This exercise is helpful for clients who habitually lean forward when sitting and freeze in this posture. If we have already practiced this *asana*, we can remind them that they can decide when they want to sit up straight again, and that they can sit up straight to once again curve their back—which means going into a Cat–Cow movement. In this way, clients get a sense of empowerment because they decide to go into the posture and get back out of it again.

VARIATIONS OF CAT–COW POSE
Bigger movements; self-touch.

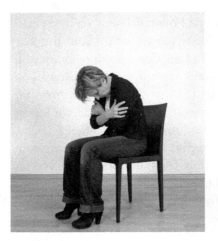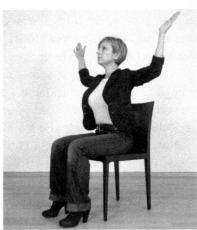

I would now like to invite you to do an *asana* that links the breath and movement, which you are already familiar with from the Cat-Cow *asana*... Take your time to find a comfortable starting position... When you are ready, cross your arms in front of your chest and bend your head and torso slightly. Put your hands on your elbows or place them further up on your arms. You decide what feels good and how much you want to bend your upper body...

As you inhale, move your upper body into an upright position... open your arms and spread them. You also control the degree of this movement... You can just slightly move your arms to the side or open them wider... How high you want to lift your arms and the pace of your movement is entirely up to you. Go ahead and try out the different variations while we move in the breath rhythm...

PRACTICE TIP: I comment on the movements of the clients like this: "When you breathe in, cross your arms in front of your chest. When you breathe out, open your arms as wide as you wish. You move in your own rhythm and at your own speed. You also decide whether you even want to move in time with your breath. Perhaps another rhythm feels more appropriate to you at the moment."

I use this *asana*, which emphasizes both opening when sitting up straight and tightness when leaning, as the progression of the Cat–Cow when clients have mastered the simple forward bend and backbend. At the same time, this *asana* brings about a natural self-touch and changes the emotional experiencing.

A female client described her reaction: "When I lean forward, I make myself very small. On the one hand, this is very frightening and not very easy for me. But holding on to my arms makes it easier. When I sit up straight and open upward, I feel very vulnerable and exposed to others, but also courageous and tall. That I can go back is a good thought, as is the idea that I can decide on and vary the movement on my own. So the fear doesn't become overwhelming."

A second female client experienced this *asana* in an entirely different way: "When I hold my upper arms, I feel bad. This is unpleasant and oppressive." We found a tolerable position for her hands: She crossed them in front of her chest.

ACTIVATING SEATED POSES
BACKBEND

Opening the chest; vulnerability; less protection; but also sitting up straight and taking up more space.

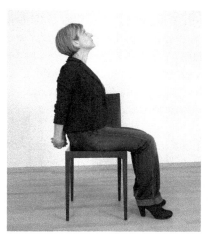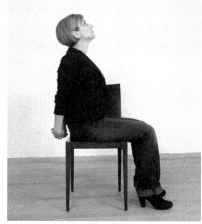

For a backbend, it's best to sit sideways on the chair so that the back of the chair is not in the way. To stabilize your lumbar spine, put your hands in the area of your kidneys and pull your navel inward… When you are ready, open your chest by pulling back your shoulders…and move your sternum upward... Just bend your neck very gently. You can keep your eyes open or closed...whatever you prefer... You decide how far back you want to lean and stretch your chest muscles... Do the backbend in the way that is appropriate for you at the moment... You may notice a stretch of your chest muscles...or the muscles in your shoulders. Perhaps you would like to direct your attention to your hands, which support your back...or to your feet, which carry less weight...

You may discover entirely different sensations as you allow your attention to stay on your body. You can also focus on the breath movement...observe how the breath movement in your chest area or belly makes itself felt... Perhaps you would like to spend more time in the backbend...or release the pose at your own pace... Take your time... And perhaps you now have the desire to move your shoulders a little and circle them—whatever feels appropriate to you. See what your body is signaling at the present moment.

VARIATIONS OF BACKBEND

If you would like to put a bit more intensity into the backbend, interlace your fingers behind your back... You have now several possibilities.

You can open your shoulders and allow your shoulder blades to come together...and perhaps stay here for a moment or longer... Perhaps you sense a strong stretch in your chest muscles... Check time and again to see whether you are still breathing and how you now notice the movement of the breath...

Another possibility is to pull your arms down a bit...and also stretch the arm muscles... You can also try out both variations or perhaps find another possibility for doing this *asana*...

PRACTICE TIP: Opening the chest can trigger a feeling of defenselessness. How wide the movement can be and how long it can be tolerated is determined by the clients themselves. I remind them of this time and again. I often only offer the backbend when clients have had experiences with the dynamic variations of the Cat–Cow Pose. Since they are already familiar with the position of the backbend by this time, they also "know" how to come back out of it when it gets to be too much. This is important since sitting up straight and therefore taking up more space not only evokes feelings of empowerment, but may possibly also cause fear. If exposure had previously been dangerous for clients, sitting up straight probably won't awaken any positive feelings at first. But if it's gradually tolerated, this posture can become a resource.

DYNAMIC SIDE BEND
Learning to tolerate faster powerful breathing; promoting presence in the here and now.

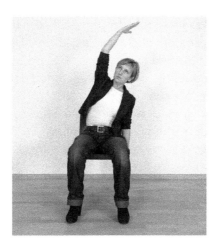

(We start in Mountain Pose.) We can bring some dynamic into play by lifting both arms, if you like... You can stretch your arms up vertically... or also hold them slightly bent...whatever feels appropriate... When you are ready, bend a little to the left... You can try out how far... Perhaps you notice the weight of your arms...or the muscles in your shoulder area...or possibly even something entirely different...

Now we'll begin moving the upper body rhythmically by alternating from the right to the left... As you do this, synchronize the movement with your breath...or choose a different rhythm... The rhythm of the movement can be faster or slower...powerful or gentle... You can also decide whether you want to breathe through your mouth or nose... Both are fine... If you like, you can try how it feels to combine powerful breathing with an active movement. We can accelerate the movement... You decide on your pace...and powerfully inhale and exhale the breath.

If you like, we can do the movements three to four more times... and then allow your arms to lower at your own pace...and allow yourself a moment to notice the sensation… You may feel a change in your breathing rhythm…how it becomes slower…perhaps a sense of warmth… It may be that you don't notice any of this—this is completely fine. Perceiving nothing is also a perception.

PRACTICE TIP: Strenuous static postures often result in people holding their breath. Dynamic *asanas* counteract this tendency since breathing is part of the exercise. A faster or more powerful breath can be a trigger, which also applies to the sound of the breath. This *asana* should be introduced carefully by starting with slow movements and a soft breath. As has been described, both can be intensified over time.

Clients frequently pull up their shoulders when they do this. When we observe this, it's advisable to consciously raise and lower our shoulders several times with the clients. This will gradually give them a feeling for where they position their shoulders, and that they can perhaps also relax and lower them a bit in everyday life. We do not point this out to them and correct the "wrong" posture.

STAFF POSE
Actively sensing the entire body; sitting up straight; perceiving strength.

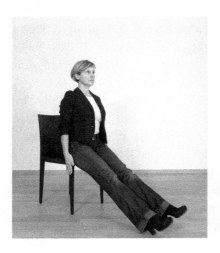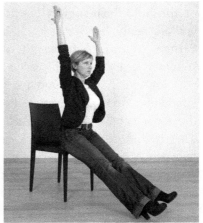

For Staff Pose, it's helpful to slide a bit forward and get comfortable at the edge of the chair. Take the time to find a good and stable position. If you now activate your abdominal muscles to support your lumbar spine...and allow your spinal column to grow taller... I would like to invite you to stay in this position for a moment and determine whether your breath is still flowing...and if it has faltered, start breathing again... When you are ready, you have a choice between two options. You can place your arms at your side or...stretch your arms and hands upward... Perhaps the activity allows you to sense your muscles in your hands and arms, perhaps also your shoulder muscles...

Now I would like to invite you to stretch out your legs to the front...and stay in this position for a moment to observe what has changed in your body...perhaps the sensations in the back leg muscles... You may also feel changes in your abdominal muscles...or something entirely different...

Take your time in exploring the *asana* and finding out which muscles have become active...as well as where and how you feel the exertion... You can become even more active by pulling up your toes...and perhaps you notice a stretch on the back side of your leg muscles...or if completely different sensations arise... You can bring movement to the *asana* by pulling up your toes...and then stretching them again...in your own rhythm...

If you want to be even more active, you can raise your stretched right leg and think of the activated abdominal muscles, which support your lumbar spine... How high you take your leg...and how long you want to stay in the *asana*...is up to you. One possibility for feeling the muscle in your thigh is to place a hand on this muscle... But also think briefly about your breath and let it flow...

I am now releasing this *asana*, and you can follow me...or just stay in the posture as long as you like... Once you have brought your leg and arms down again... I would like to invite you to determine whether your right leg feels any different from the left...or whether you notice how the exertion in your leg or even in your arms and shoulders has decreased... By letting the muscles relax and recuperate, this moment of calmness also allows your entire body to recover.

PRACTICE TIP: Stretching out the legs can be a relief when clients notice that their legs and feet are very tense while sitting. Since it addresses many muscles in the body, Staff Pose is well suited for getting a sense of the entire body.

CHAIR POSITION—POWERFUL POSE
Sense of empowerment.

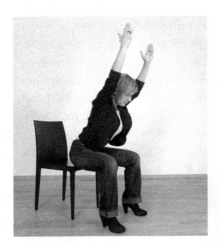 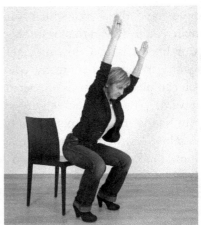

For this powerful *asana*, you should slide forward to the edge of the chair and find a secure footing on the floor... Position your feet a bit wider than hip width... Take the time to make yourself comfortable... When you are ready, I would like to invite you to raise your arms to shoulder height...or stretch them even higher... You decide how you would like to practice this *asana*... As always, activate your abdominal muscles.

In a further step, pretend that you want to get up from the chair... so that you get into a position where you float slightly above the chair... It's easy to hold your breath during exertion, so I would like to invite you to check this...and allow your breath to keep flowing in case it has stopped... As long as you continue to breathe in a regular way, your body knows that everything is okay. I invite you to focus on your thigh muscles... You can get a more distinct feeling for the muscle activity in your quadriceps if you place your hands on them...and then stretch upward again... You may feel an especially intense exertion in your arms and shoulders...or at some other place in your body... Perhaps we can remain in this posture for a few more breaths... I will count backward from 4 to 1... But you decide when it's enough and allow yourself to sink back down on your chair at your own pace...

It's easy to come up into a standing position from Chair Position.

PRACTICE TIP: If clients tend to dissociate or freeze in these strenuous static positions, you can turn any of the static exercises into dynamic ones. In Chair Position, you can suggest to clients that they slightly move up and down, synchronize this movement with the breath, or also synchronously move their arms with the breath, as in the Sun Breath (see Chapter 14). We always remind them of breathing and the breath *movement*.

BOAT POSE
Sensing the power in the center; varying the intensity of the *asana*.

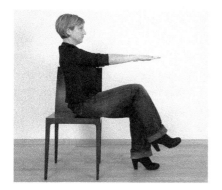 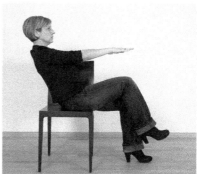

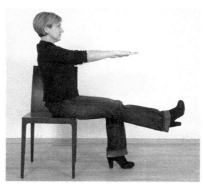

For Boat Pose, once again sit sideways on the chair so that your back is free... In this *asana*, it is important to activate the navel point so that your lumbar spine is stabilized... Take your time to get comfortable... and perhaps you will also notice the contact that your sit bones have with the contact points and areas on the chair... As soon as you are ready, raise your right foot... Perhaps you already feel how the muscles in your belly and legs are working... If you like, place one hand on your thigh or belly...and then alternately raise your foot and put it back down on the floor again... Perhaps you feel the muscle tensing and relaxation more clearly in this way...

At the moment, I'm sensing the activity of my abdominal muscles when I raise my leg... Briefly check to see whether you are still breathing... This gives your body the signal that everything is fine. Now you can stretch out your arms to the front and parallel to the floor... Perhaps you sense a change in your abdominal muscles... possibly also in your shoulder and arm muscles...

If you are in the mood for more intensity, pull your leg closer to your chest... Perhaps you notice the activity in your abdominal muscles...but perhaps also your back muscles...or your arms... You decide how intensively you want to do this *asana* and how long you want to hold it... I will count backwards from 4 to 1...and I invite you to get out of this *asana* at your own pace... But you can just as well go into a neutral position at any time... Once you have come back to it again...you can take a moment to compare the right side of the body with the left side... Perhaps there is a difference... You may possibly observe while you pause how the exertion leaves your muscles...

If you agree with this, I would now like to repeat the course of the exercise with the left leg. You can do the *asana* on this side just like on the other... However, you can also do it entirely differently... Since the halves of the body are never entirely the same, it can be interesting to compare both sides of the body with each other... Perhaps there is a difference...

VARIATIONS OF BOAT POSE

You can also lean further back...but always make sure that your navel is pulled in... You may feel the activity more intensely in your abdominal muscles.

Instead of pulling your leg to your chest, you can also stretch out your leg parallel to the floor... As you do this, you may especially notice the weight of your leg... You can check again to see if your breath is still flowing. In case it has stopped, start the flow of your breath again. If you would like to, pull your toes toward yourself...and then stretch them away from you again...and notice what changes in your leg muscles...

PRACTICE TIP: This *asana* offers many variation possibilities. Depending on how you do it, making little changes can be more or less strenuous. Together with your clients you can find out whether they have a habit of choosing the more strenuous variations and how it feels when they do not go to their own limits or when they think that they are not capable of anything and give up immediately. At such moments, it is possible to recognize beliefs, but we do not discuss them. Instead, we strive for fresh experiences in the exploration of something new.

TRIANGLE POSE

Flexibility and stretching; opening the chest—which is less "dangerous" for some clients than pulling back both of the shoulders and arms at the same time.

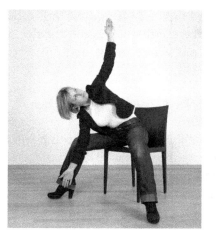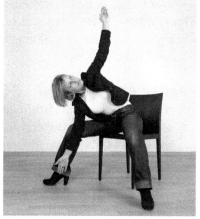

When doing Triangle Pose, it's easier if you place your feet a bit more than hip-width apart so that you have enough space for the movement... When you have found a good position for your feet... I invite you to place your right forearm above your right knee...and then take a moment to get comfortable in this pose... Once you are ready, stretch your left arm upward... You control the intensity of the *asanas* by deciding how wide your twist should be...and how much you would like to stretch your arm... Your gaze can be straight ahead...or directed up to your hand above you... This is your decision. Stay in Triangle Pose for a moment and observe which muscles you especially notice—whether due to the stretching and extending in the arm, shoulder, or chest muscles… Or perhaps you notice the weight of your arms or upper body…

VARIATIONS OF TRIANGLE POSE

You now have various possibilities. You can stretch your left arm further up and back…also intensify the twist… Another possibility is to place your right forearm on the inside of your lower left leg…with your hand at the height of your calf…or your ankle… And perhaps you notice a change in the flow of your breath…or through the intensity of the twists to your left side…or something completely different… Your gaze can continue to be upward or straight ahead.

You control how much strength you use and the length of time that you want to stay in the *asana*… I will count backwards from 4 and invite you to end the *asana* then or immediately… After you release the *asana*, take your time…so that your muscles can recuperate and relax. You may notice that the left and right side feels differently after Triangle Pose… Or you sense how the exertion leaves the muscles… Let's give the muscles a moment of rest before we go into this *asana* on the other side.

PRACTICE TIP: After you have practiced Triangle Pose, you can risk trying an *asana* that requires more opening of the chest such as a slight backbend, possibly with the hands interlaced behind the back. Or suggest opening the arms upward or to the side in Mountain Pose. After the half-sided opening through Triangle Pose, it is frequently less of a problem to open the chest further.

STANDING POSES

Standing poses are suited for grounding, getting a sense of standing on solid ground, experiencing stability, and developing a feeling for our own center. It is also sometimes important to assume a different perspective: We "grow" when we stand and feel perhaps a bit more "grown up."

When in the standing *asanas we can frequently observe*:

- knees are locked

- shoulders are pulled upward

- the chest is sunken

- the upper back is stooped

- clients stand with a sway back

- the arms hang down feebly

- a breath movement can hardly be detected.

These "mistakes" are not addressed and corrected. We solely determine what the posture patterns are and include variations—by making suggestions—with which clients can gradually have new experiences. The posture and movement patterns of clients have developed for a certain reason. They have often been a part of their defense strategy for decades. If we force a change of these movement and posture patterns, we are in danger of overwhelming the clients.

As an example of how to deal with posture patterns, we observe that the clients tensely stand across from us and have their shoulders pulled up. When practicing an *asana*, we can suggest to the clients that they pull up their shoulders and lower them. They can repeat this a few times at their own pace, if they like.

BASIC STANDING POSES
MOUNTAIN POSE
Basic pose and starting position for standing *asanas*; grounding while simultaneously growing tall.

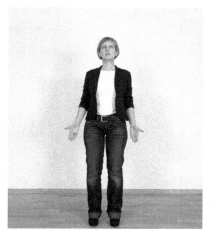 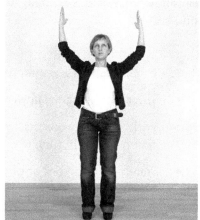

I would like to invite you to assume Mountain Pose standing up. When you are ready, feel your contact with the floor and the sensations in your feet... You may feel the weight of your body...or notice your foot muscles. You can activate your foot muscles by moving your toes... spreading them...or curling them. Perhaps you notice the texture of the floor as you do this...or the temperature of your feet or the points where they touch the floor. In order to feel your feet, it can be helpful to move them back and forth on the floor.

If you let your attention wander to your knees...they may be stretched or slightly bent. Here as well, I would like to invite you to try out how it feels when your knees are bent a little...and then stretch them out straight again... If you repeat this a few times, you may feel your leg muscles or knee joints...or notice something in another area of your body. For the yoga poses, it is good to not lock your knees completely so that they stay flexible. Be sure to also think about your abdominal muscles... When you activate them, you also support your lower back. This activation can also have an effect on your breath... You may discover that your breath is no longer flowing quite as deeply...but when you focus on your costal ribs...you may feel more movement here... Your attention can now wander further up to your shoulders... You may feel the muscles around your shoulders and upper back. You can consciously pull your shoulders up...and lower them again, at your own pace. If you like, you can repeat the movement a few times. It's also fine to just notice your shoulders and determine where they are. As we now complete Mountain Pose, our eyes are directed straight ahead and palms are facing forward. You can also allow your hands to hang down loosely at your side, however you like.

VARIATIONS OF MOUNTAIN POSE
There are many variations to improve interoception. Here is a selection:

- Stretching the arms upward.

- With little movements to the right, left, back, or front, in search of equilibrium.

- Standing on tiptoes or on the heels.

- Switching from the toes to the heels.

- Bending the knees and stretching them again.

- Turning the arms so that the palms face backward and return to the front again.

- Pulling up the shoulders and then lowering or circling them.

- Moving the arms up and down at the side or in front.

- Tilting or circling the head to the right and left in small movements.

- Slightly raising the head (but avoiding hyperextension of the cervical spine) and tilting it.

TREE POSE
Finding balance; concentration.

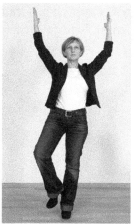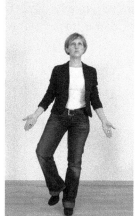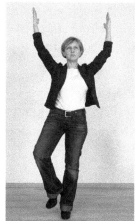

An *asana* to improve your sense of balance is Tree Pose. You can use a chair as an aid by holding on to its back...or freely vary this *asana*. As soon as you have anchored yourself on the floor...and have assumed a secure position...shift your weight to your right leg and take a moment to be aware of this leg. You may already sense activity in your leg and feet muscles due to the weight shift...and you may possibly also notice a difference between right and left. When you are ready, shift your weight entirely to your right foot...and place your left foot on your right ankle... You can perhaps notice the little movements that your leg muscles make to keep you in balance... You determine where you want to place your arms...on the back of the chair...next to your body...or stretched above your head. In this posture, it is also a good idea to activate your abdominal muscles...

To keep your balance, it can be helpful if you fix your eyes on a steady point on the floor about a yard in front of you... You may notice that you are holding your breath... If so, start breathing again. You can direct your attention to your standing leg or some of part of your body...whatever you prefer.

You can stay even longer in the *asana* or end the pose.

Before we change sides... I invite you to notice the difference in both legs... Perhaps you notice the fading tension in your right leg...or have entirely different sensations. If you allow your body a little rest and time to recuperate, you may also notice that your breath movements and breath have become deeper.

PRACTICE TIP: Tree Pose requires concentration and inner balance. Once we have practiced Tree Pose, some clients notice that they are not always balanced equally well. They register that it can help them to always come back to the "center" and find their equilibrium.

CALMING STANDING POSES
GENTLE SIDE BEND
Grounding; stretching.

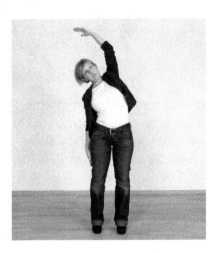

If you like, we can bring a bit of stretch into play for Mountain Pose. If you agree, I invite you to raise your right arm... Let your left arm hang down loosely... You can stretch your right arm...or keep it slightly bent—whatever feels appropriate to you... When you are ready...bend your upper body a little to the left. While bending, you may notice a stretch of your side muscles... You may feel the muscles between your costal ribs... You may notice the weight of your arm... When you observe your breath...you may notice that your breath movement has changed. If you want more intensity...bring your left hand to your right and stretch both arms upward.

Now lower your right arm or both arms...by giving your muscles a moment of rest...check whether you feel a difference between the right and left side... Perhaps you notice that one side has been stretched...but not the other... Or you may not sense any of this...or something totally different. This is completely okay.

When you are ready...change sides... I invite you to stretch your left arm upward... Here as well, you decide on the position of your arms.

PRACTICE TIP: If you want to turn the static *asana* into a dynamic one, invite the clients to alternate moving to the right and the left. Once again, this exercise can be synchronized with the breath.

VARIATIONS OF CALMING STANDING POSES

- Swing the upper body back and forth like a pendulum.

- Let the arms passively swing back and forth with the pendulum movement.

- Do circling movements with the upper body or entire body.

FORWARD BEND STANDING UP

Like the seated form (see above), the forward bend can also be done in standing. Stand with the feet wider apart than hip width. Clients decide for themselves how far the straddle should be.

VARIATIONS OF FORWARD BEND STANDING UP

- Arms, hands, and head hang loosely.

- Let the arms swing back and forth.

- Do yes/no movements with the head.

- Bend and stretch the knees.

- Move toward the right leg in the straddle. Stay there for a little while, and stretch—then do the same on the left.

ACTIVATING STANDING POSES
DOWNWARD DOG POSE (ON A CHAIR)/ THREE-LEGGED DOG POSE
Powerful posture; interrupting dissociation.

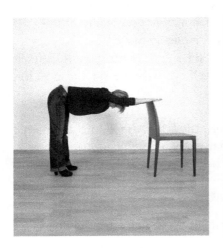 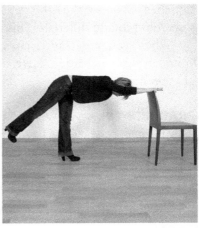

I would like to introduce an *asana*...a controlled forward bend in standing...Downward Dog Pose. If you want to try this out...place your chair so that your hands can touch the backrest with outstretched arms when you bend forward...

As soon as you are in position...and standing with your feet hip-width apart...you may want to check this by looking at your feet... and also focus on your legs... And as soon as you have a secure position, stretch your arms upward...bend forward...until you reach the back of the chair... If you like, you can do a few movements with your spinal column...such as the Cat–Cow...and coordinate them with your breath...

One variation is to align your upper body horizontally in a straight line that is parallel to the floor...breathe through your mouth or nose—whatever feels best... You may notice the movement of your breathing...or your stretched arm muscles...or your back muscles as they hold you. Another possibility is to pull your right arm forward and lengthen your right side as a result. But you can also stretch both of your arms forward at the same time… To do this, push the chair away from you a bit so that your entire back is extended…and notice what changes in your body as you do this.

VARIATIONS OF THREE-LEGGED DOG POSE

You can intensify the pose by raising one stretched leg… You decide how high you would like to lift this leg. Activate your abdominal muscles as you do this.

PRACTICE TIP: Downward Dog Pose is well suited for interrupting dissociation. I choose this variation when the "real" Downward Dog Pose (see earlier) isn't possible.

WARRIOR I POSE

Power and strength; interrupting dissociation.

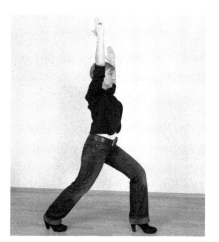 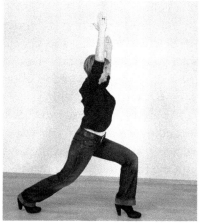

The Warrior Poses are powerful standing *asanas*. For Warrior I Pose, we take a big step forward with the right foot… You decide how big this step should be… If you like, stay in this pose for a moment…find your balance and direct your attention to the muscle activity in your body…or focus on your breath. For the next step, I invite you to bend your front knee… The left leg stays stretched… To keep your knee joint safe, please make sure that your right knee is positioned vertically above your ankle. You can also put it behind the ankle... Perhaps you would like to take a look at the position of your knee? (If the knee is too far forward, this harms the knee joint. See below.)

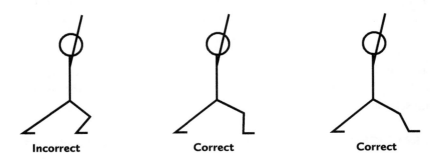

Incorrect   **Correct**   **Correct**

You can control the intensity of the *asanas* by going into a stronger or less pronounced bend... Experiment to see how it is appropriate for you... In this powerful posture, we often hold our breath...and perhaps you would like to focus on your breath for a moment... and check whether it is still flowing...or has faltered. Now you can raise your arms...

You have various possibilities: You can keep your arms bent... or stretched. You can also decide to what extent you would like to open your chest...by bringing your elbows more or less to the back. I would like to invite you to observe what you notice in your body— warmth, exertion, stretching, movement, or weight...

At every moment, you control the intensity of the *asana*... depending on whether you want to go more or less deeply into it... whatever works for you right now. If you like, you can stay in the pose with me for a few more breaths...or end it now and come out of this *asana* at your own pace... For example, by stretching your front leg... then letting your arms come down...and finally bringing your legs closer together again.

You can come out of the *asana* in your own personal way. Perhaps you would like to shake out your arms and legs...and then allow your muscles a bit of rest and relaxation. You may feel some changes in your muscles...such as an easing of the tension or a sense of heaviness... or maybe not. Should your breath or heartbeat have sped up a bit, you may notice that both have now calmed down again... If you like, rest for a moment before we change sides.

PRACTICE TIP: Just like Downward Dog Pose, I primarily suggest the Warrior *asanas* to clients who habitually fall into a flaccid immobility. In this case, include them in the clients' home program. Clients usually feel that the Warrior Poses are empowering postures that remind them of their power and strength. Since they train both balance and strength, many muscles are involved in these poses and give clients a sense of their entire body

WARRIOR II POSE
Power and strength; interrupting dissociation.

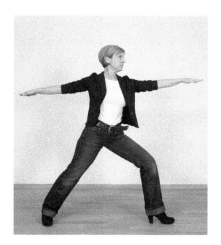 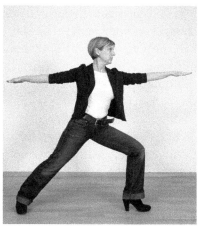

For this powerful *asana*, we go into a wide straddle. Take a moment and check to see what you now notice in your legs…hips…or somewhere else in your body… When you are ready…turn your right foot outward so that the tip of the foot points to the right side… To stabilize your lumbar spine, please activate your abdominal muscles again. Now bend your right knee…but keep your left leg stretched… Remember the knee position of Warrior I Pose. Take a look at your knee to make sure that it is located behind or vertically above your ankle… Take your time…and feel your way into the pose…and when you are ready…observe what is happening in your body: movements… breathing…stretching…the activity in your muscles… You control the intensity of the *asana* at all times…by deciding how gently…or intensely you would like to go into the bend…

When you are ready for the next step...spread both your arms at the height of your shoulders and parallel to the floor...or just as high or low as you feel like...and hold your arms in this position... Next, turn your upper body to the front...direct your gaze into the distance over your bent knee... Now you have various possibilities for bringing movement into this *asana*... For example, by swinging your arms with the rhythm of your breath...inhale high...exhale low...

If you would like to stay a bit longer in the *asana*, simply stay as long as is appropriate for you...or come out of the *asana* at your own pace... For example, by stretching your front leg and allowing your arms to lower... Perhaps you would like to shake out your arms and legs and then allow your muscles some relaxation. You may feel some changes in your muscles as you do this...a decreasing of the tension or a heaviness...or perhaps none of these or something completely different... Your breath or heartbeat may now normalize again...

If you like, stay in this state of calmness—which gives your body the necessary recuperation—for a moment before we change sides.

TABLE POSE AND DOWNWARD DOG POSE
Change of perspective; interrupting dissociation.

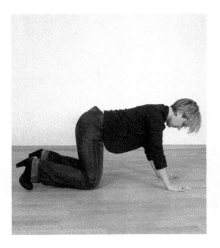 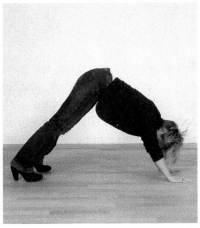

I would like to show you another powerful exercise... We can go into Downward Dog Pose from Table Pose...but you can also push up out of a crouch (see "Variations") into Downward Dog Pose... Let's try out both variations...so that you can discover which one is better for you...

We set up Table Pose...by going on to all fours and placing the hands beneath the shoulders... Feel free to check your hands and arms by looking at them... You may feel the weight that rests on your hands...or the floor beneath your hands ... Your knees are beneath your hip joints... It also helps here to check the position by looking at it... You may need padding under your knees...a blanket or a pillow...

When you are ready, pull in your navel in the direction of your lumbar spine...and then push your bottom upward... Your legs are stretched...or slightly bent, whatever is possible for you...your heels are pulling in the direction of the floor... It may feel more pleasant to place a blanket under your heels so your heels make contact... (A blanket can be offered at this point.) You can either allow your head to hang down loosely...or you can look toward your knees... You may sense the weight on your hands...or the strength that you must exert in your shoulders to hold the *asana*... There may even be a pulling in your calves and the backs of your knees... I suggest that we stay in this pose for another three to four breaths...and then come out of it... You can end the *asana* at any time...or even stay in it a bit longer.

You can come out of the *asana* in your own way...or return to Table Pose, which is the all-fours position...and from there, you can sit on your heels...to pause for a moment... Or you can also go from the all-fours position into a crouch and come into an upright position from there... Now give your muscles a moment to relax... And you may possibly feel how the tension in your legs is easing...or your shoulder muscles are relaxing...

VARIATIONS

Let's get into the crouch together... Put your hands as far in front of your feet as possible... When you are ready, push your bottom upward...stretch out your legs...and "walk" with your hands...so that there is more distance between your feet and hands.

PRACTICE TIP: I use Downward Dog Pose when clients dissociate and I want to show them a possibility for quickly finding their way back to the here and now. It is best to practice Downward Dog Pose within the framework of a "neutral" yoga sequence so that extensive explanations are not necessary at this point. When clients are in a dissociated state, we can no longer reach them.

Downward Dog Pose can be assumed from a crouch. For people who have been sexually traumatized, a pose in which the genitals and buttocks are not protected represents a trigger. When these clients first start practicing, these are not suitable positions, so the crouch can be a good variation in these cases.

14

PRANAYAMA

When we want to train clients in *pranayama*, it's helpful to become familiar with some details of breathing, breath musculature, and the various types and spaces of breath. This knowledge enables us to instruct *pranayama* exercises in a more specific way.

PRANAYAMA IN ANATOMICAL TERMS

We tend to breathe without being aware of it. It is a process that works automatically most of the time: We don't need to attend to it and leave its control up to our body. Yet we still have the freedom to make decisions about our breath. We can change its depth and frequency at any time, as well as hold our breath for a certain amount of time. The yogis recognized the value of influencing the breath and emphasized the physical and psychological use of breath control in their ancient writings (cf. Coulter 2009; Fuchs 2007).

Seen in a physiological sense, breathing is the inflow and outflow of air in the lungs, which is shown by the movement of the abdominal and chest cavity. During breathing, both body cavities change their form—but with an important difference: The abdominal cavity only changes its form, but not its volume. It arches to the outside since the diaphragm pushes down the inner organs as it lowers. Then it pulls back again. By contrast, the chest cavity changes both its form and its volume. When we inhale, the rib cage expands so that the air is pressed into the lungs through the atmospheric pressure. This process is reversed during relaxed calm exhalation. The chest cavity contracts and the air passively flows out of it.

The chest cavity and abdominal cavity change their form in a three-dimensional way: from top to bottom, left to right, and front to back. The most important respiratory muscle is the diaphragm, which causes this displacement in the chest and belly. It separates the chest area from the abdomen, has the shape of an umbrella, and is anchored to the skeleton in three places: at the lower end of the sternum, edge of the rib cage, and front of the lumbar spine. The diaphragm is not attached anywhere at the "top" since it actually ends within itself in a flat horizontal roof—the tendon plate.

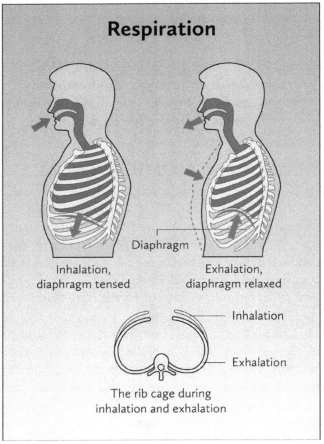

RESPIRATION AND THE DIAPHRAGM (© ROB3000 – FOTOLIA.COM)

The muscle activity of the diaphragm is generally linked with abdominal breathing: The belly arches outward during inhalation and flattens again during exhalation. Yet the diaphragm is no less involved in the chest breathing. When the intercostal musculature relaxes, its simultaneous contraction results in an expansion of the rib cage.

The most important respiratory accessory muscles are the intercostal muscles and the abdominal muscles. The former are divided into the external and internal intercostal musculature. They play a main role in the movement of the rib cage. The external muscles lift the rib cage and extend the ribs to support inhalation; for a complete exhalation, the internal muscles pull it downward and inward. In contrast to the subjective perception, the distances remain constant since the ribs just shift against each other.

The movement and expansion of the rib cage can only take place when the intercostal muscles are relaxed. For abdominal breathing, it's very important to have a relaxed abdominal wall. Tight or tense abdominal muscles make it more difficult to arch the belly when inhaling. But this also applies: Since the abdominal muscles are directly connected with the rib cage, their state of tension has a direct influence on the flexibility of the intercostal muscles and on the chest breathing as a result.

Abdominal breathing is often propagated as the "right" type of breathing and the chest breathing is seen as "wrong" since only the former is mistakenly considered to be diaphragmatic breathing. As explained above, the diaphragm is involved in both cases. The belly can also be arched to the outside without an inhalation occurring. One example of this is the paradoxical breathing pattern (more on this below).

PRANAYAMA IN PRACTICAL TERMS
TYPES OF BREATHING

As in the *asana* practice, the use of *pranayama* in the trauma therapy means that we study the individual forms with our clients. But before we explore the breath with them, we should first take a look at the breath as such, the breath in various emotional states, and our own breathing pattern. It's important to first discover how the various forms of breathing affect us.

The different forms of breathing are: shallow chest breathing, paradoxical breathing, relaxed abdominal breathing, energizing chest breathing, and breathing in an emotional stupor. The exercises marked with * are solely intended for exploring your own interoception.

Shallow chest breathing

Shallow chest breathing is fast and intermittent. In this type of breathing, just the upper part of the rib cage is lifted. The abdominal wall and lower ribs do not move.

EXERCISE: SHALLOW CHEST BREATHING

Inhale and exhale quickly for 20 to 30 times by just moving the upper part of the rib cage, which is the collarbone area. Pay attention to the effects of this breathing pattern.

After doing this exercise, an unsettled feeling will probably arise and you will have the irresistible urge to take a few deep breaths. In this type of chest breathing, you will feel like you are constantly somewhat out of breath since the major portion of the air is drawn into the upper lobe of the lungs. Since the lower parts of the lungs have the best blood supply, less oxygen gets into the blood as a result.

Paradoxical breathing

The trigger for paradoxical breathing is a shock situation. During inhalation, the abdominal wall moves inward. The intercostal muscles raise the rib cage and pull up the relaxed diaphragm and the abdominal organs. During exhalation, the belly arches outward because the rib cage relaxes.

*EXERCISE: PARADOXICAL BREATHING

Imagine that you are expecting a warm shower and have ice-cold water poured over you instead! This is how you can easily simulate paradoxical breathing and feel its effects.

Paradoxical breathing prepares us for a fight-or-flight reaction and causes an immediate adrenaline rush. Many people breathe like this for their entire lifetime, which keeps their sympathetic nervous system in a state of constant arousal. This breathing pattern—which stimulates the sympathetic nervous system even more intensely than chest breathing—can be observed in many trauma clients.

RELAXED ABDOMINAL BREATHING

Relaxed abdominal breathing only succeeds with relaxed abdominal muscles; it's not possible when they are tense. In abdominal breathing, the rib cage hardly moves and the lower abdomen arches slightly forward and back. The intercostal muscles are only active in so far as they must keep the rib cage stable when the diaphragm is pulled downward. The head and throat are pulled back slightly during inhalation.

*EXERCISE: RELAXED ABDOMINAL BREATHING

Remove any constricting clothing and sit upright on a chair. At the start, let your breath flow and observe your breathing pattern. Relax your abdominal wall completely. Now pay attention to the movements in your body and the effect that the abdominal breathing has on your inner state.

The two critical moments during breathing are the transitions between inhaling and exhaling or between exhaling and inhaling. It's helpful to imagine a circle or, even better, an ellipse, in order not to breathe in a jerky or uneven way during the transitions. It takes a bit of practice to make the transitions gentle.

For the sake of completeness, here is a description of the energizing chest breathing to counter the misunderstanding that every type of chest breathing is "wrong."

ENERGIZING CHEST BREATHING

Energizing chest breathing plays a major role in yoga since it widens the chest area. It ensures adequate oxygen when the abdominal muscles are activated and relaxed abdominal breathing is not possible. In certain positions, such as a forward bend, the abdominal area cannot expand. The best way to do the energizing chest breathing is by sticking out the chest. The belly and diaphragm remain relatively stable. The sternum moves upward and to the front like a pump handle, and the intercostal musculature extends.

*EXERCISE: ENERGIZING CHEST BREATHING

Interlace your hands behind your head and bend back a little. When inhaling, be sure that you have a maximum expansion of the chest. This allows you to most clearly feel the movement of your sternum and intercostal musculature.

In contrast to shallow chest breathing, you receive abundant air and oxygen. This is an effective remedy in situations where you are tired and lose concentration. Incidentally, this type of breathing allows you to most clearly feel the three-dimensional movement of your rib cage.

For most trauma clients, this exercise is not suitable—at least not at the start of the *pranayama* practice. However, it can clearly show you the anatomical aspects and refine your own interoception.

BREATHING IN AN EMOTIONAL STUPOR

If you would like to understand how clients feel when they are frozen in the emotional stupor of their trauma, visualize the postural patterns and breathing patterns so that you can literally experience them in your own body. I recommend exploring your own breathing in the state of frozen fear.

*EXERCISE: BREATHING IN AN EMOTIONAL STUPOR

Act as if you were frightened to the core and then stay in this posture and continue to breathe—as well as you can. What do you feel or notice?

You will probably register the following: Your shoulders are drawn upward and the intercostal muscles pull your rib cage outward and up. At the same time, your diaphragm and abdominal muscles are tensed. The movement of your chest and abdominal area is restricted. Your breathing becomes shallow and blocks breathing deep into your belly, as well as a flexible expansion of the rib cage. You hardly get any air.

We can assume that trauma clients use shallow chest breathing. We occasionally see a few deep breaths that transport the air in the lower parts of the lungs, which have better circulation, and therefore ensure a somewhat adequate supply of oxygen in the body. In addition to shallow chest breathing, you can also notice paradoxical breathing. Both show the embodied fright and frozen fear. They sustain these feelings since breathing patterns have a direct correlation with the nervous system.

GOALS OF BREATH CONTROL

Like the *asanas*, breath control helps us to investigate interoceptive processes. However, it has an additional aspect: A direct influence on the nervous system. Breath control should be introduced gradually for it to have successful and positive effects, so let's take a closer look at this process.

The somatic nervous system controls the skeletal musculature and all conscious perceptions such as sight, hearing, the tactile sense, etc. The autonomic nervous system regulates the autonomic body functions such as the heartbeat, sweat production, hormone release, digestion, and elimination. Both systems are involved in respiration.

BREATHING—AN EQUALLY DELIBERATE AND UNCONSCIOUS ACT

The somatic activity of the skeletal muscles can be deliberately controlled by the cerebral cortex and therefore changed by it. This fact is important for *pranayama* since we want to influence the breathing through the respiratory musculature.

We do not usually influence breathing deliberately. It is controlled by the respiratory centers in the brain stem, which are subcortical structures that dictate a simple rhythm. However, the "higher" structures are capable of interrupting or smoothing this flow. For example, the breath halts or becomes irregular when we are agitated. If we notice how our breath has lost its rhythm, we can deliberately "smooth it out." This process of becoming aware and having an influence on the breath is the theme of *pranayama*, the control of the breath in yoga.

As we know, the autonomic nervous system consists of the sympathetic and the parasympathetic branches. The sympathetic nervous system prepares the body for dangerous situations (fight or flight), and the parasympathetic portion is responsible for the functioning of the inner organs, as well as for the ability to relax. It plays an important role in social interactions and is decisively responsible for the shut-down in hopeless situations.

The breathing patterns have a direct influence on the autonomic nervous system. A deep relaxed abdominal breathing activates the parasympathetic nervous system, which also applies to a prolonged exhalation. An accelerated breath rhythm, superficial breathing, and prolonged inhaling and holding of the air activate the sympathetic nervous system.

As described above, breath patterns are frequently formed based on embodied fear and block deep respiration. This leads to chronic overstimulation of the sympathetic nervous system, a higher pulse rate, and elevated blood pressure. In addition, intensified jumpiness and hypervigilance contribute to frequent deep inhaling and holding of the air, which also activates the sympathetic nervous system.

The paradox is that this physiological reaction that was appropriate for a previous threat has now become frozen and causes clients to remain in a never-ending state of threat and fear due to their breathing patterns. These types of breathing patterns can stimulate autonomic reactions such as panic attacks and may be accompanied by constant feelings of fear. This sets off a vicious circle that is difficult to interrupt.

In addition, relaxation—the activation of the parasympathetic nervous system—is experienced as threatening because vigilance diminishes. If we are well intentioned in asking trauma clients to relax by breathing deeply and deliberately into their belly because this has a positive effect on the parasympathetic nervous system, we can now better understand why this advice can frequently result in activation of the sympathetic nervous system and even a flashback or dissociation in some cases. Due to the tension, abdominal breathing is often not even possible, and a deep breath is linked with fright and fear.

A female client gave me the following feedback:

> When you inspired me to take a few deep breaths, I knew that deep breathing would inevitably lead me to feeling my body—and I did not want to do this at all. I panicked and was happy when you reminded me that I had the possibility of choosing my own breathing rhythm. That was my "lifesaver." After all, I didn't have to breathe deeply!

In considering the third path of survival—the immobility reaction—under the aspect of breath, it helps to summarize what happens in the nervous system. While the sympathetic nervous system continues to fire, the dorsal vagus activates. In order to prevent a cardiac death, the activation of the sympathetic nervous system is scaled back. The body becomes flaccid to protect itself against injuries that could occur through resistance. But this moment is also the last opportunity for victims to escape because an attacker is not interested in "dead" prey. The blood flow of the periphery is reduced. The breath is only superficial and hardly visible. This very quiet, hardly perceptible breath is also advantageous when people must hide from an attacker.

This breathing pattern can also take on a life of its own and just occur in the topmost apex of the lungs. This "silent breathing" is often accompanied by the physical wish of being or becoming invisible.

In the work with trauma clients, they often hold their breath during an exposure. Once the defense cascade takes its course, the following can be observed. At the moment in which people are flooded by their trauma memories and feelings, the color leaves their face, the breath is hardly perceptible, and they dissociate. Clients often say that they are afraid of fainting in this case.

PRANAYAMA PRACTICE

When practiced on a regular basis, *pranayama* automatically causes a slowing and deepening of the breathing. With an increasing consciousness for their breath, practitioners notice in which situations they breathe in a shallow way and how this affects their state of mind. They now have the possibility of returning to a natural or deepened respiration, calming their breath and themselves in the process.

Almost all yoga books write that we breathe through the nose in yoga. It's obvious that this filters, warms, and "prepares" the air to flow into the lungs. However, even just this rule can already trigger stress because clients may not be able to fulfill this requirement. So we suggest breathing through the mouth or nose and leaving the decision up to the clients (cf. Emerson and Hopper 2011).

HOW I INTRODUCE WORKING WITH *PRANAYAMA*
FOCUSING ON THE BODY

Becoming aware of their breath is a frightening idea for some clients, so we start a breath lesson by focusing on one part of the body. This can be the nose and/or tip of the nose, if clients normally breathe through it. If they breathe through the mouth and/or lips, we focus on these areas. In addition, it's advisable to mention the stream of air that flows through the nose or mouth and the coolness of the air when it flows in, as well as the warmth when it streams out.

FOCUSING ON THE BREATH MOVEMENT

If we expand our focus to the breath movement, we can ask clients to direct their attention to their ribs. This opens up the possibility of noticing a movement of the costal arch—a rising and lowering or becoming wider. We can remind them of their spinal column and sternum, where the ribs are attached. And we can mention that the sternum raises and lowers again during deep breaths. We can also lead our clients to the collarbones and shoulders. They can be encouraged to pay attention to the little movements in the chest and shoulders that accompany the breath rhythm. We address the muscles between the ribs, which are stretched and contracted, in a very functional way.

Anatomic details and terms often facilitate access to the body and lead away from emotions. Feeling something concrete such as muscles, stretching, raising and lowering, expansiveness, or movement allows a (new) relationship with the body. Something happens; there is movement and change—which is the opposite of immobility. Not too many anatomical details should be introduced at one time. As in the instructions for the *asanas*, we choose one or two possibilities and initially concentrate on them.

Quite a few clients arrive with an idea of the "wrong" and "right" ways to breathe. They often put themselves under pressure to follow a concept that was taught to them as "right." So it's important to emphasize that this is not about right or wrong when we introduce the breath. This also doesn't yet involve changing, deepening, or slowing down the breath. Pure observation is enough for the time being. Tasks that clients cannot (yet) handle impair their sense of self-worth and lead to pressure and tension.

We can also invite clients to place one hand on their belly and the other on one of their collarbones. This gesture has a calming effect, and it makes the breath movements more distinct. It also allows clients to become familiar with the effects of their breathing.

INFLUENCING THE BREATH—FIRST STEPS

If we now take a first step in the direction of influencing the breath, we can introduce this in the following way. When the client places a hand on their belly or hands on their ribs, they may be able to consciously generate more movement under their hand(s). If these first exercises are successful, we can introduce additional forms of breath control with the possibilities for *pranayama* suggested in the next section. If we want to explain the purpose of breath control, we cannot emphasize often enough that slow breathing gives the body a feeling of security and control. As a contrast, fast breathing and/or the held breath are signals for "caution, danger!" We can also observe a holding of the breath when practicing the *asanas*. As soon as people exert themselves, they automatically hold their breath. In these cases, we can remind our clients about the flow and effect of the breath when we notice it.

It is a valuable experience to have the breath flow quietly, even though tension predominates in the body due to exertion.

At the same time, it must be clear to us that these "truths" do not apply to every trauma client. For some people, a fast breath rhythm—which leaves their sympathetic nervous system "switched on"—can definitely feel appropriate. They may mistake relaxation for decreased alertness and negligence, which is why they classify it as dangerous. For sexually traumatized people, deep breathing can also mean feeling the body beneath the navel, the pelvic floor, and possibly the genitals or the buttocks—something that they have strictly attempted to avoid in the past.

We do not support the avoidance, but should deal with it in a conscious and careful way. And it must be clear to us that learning this type of breathing can take some time. So we only introduce stress-triggering breathing and postural variations when clients have built up enough containment. If we adapt the speed of our approach to the clients' possibilities, they can access these effective resources without fear and use them to influence their nervous system. Our task is to accompany them through this process since this is how they go beyond the passive survival mechanism to an active sense of liveliness. This demands our creativity in also finding suitable solutions for these clients.

PRANAYAMA EXERCISES

The following pages contain exercise instructions for the various *pranayama* techniques. As you did with the *asanas* in the previous chapter, read them, try them out, and find your own style and personal choice of words.

COHERENT BREATHING

Coherent breathing is the simplest form of breath control, in which we initially just influence the rhythm but not the type of breathing. The goal is to have an equally long inhalation and exhalation, which can have a calming effect. This exercise prepares clients for an extension of the exhalation.

EXERCISE: COHERENT BREATHING

I invite you to observe your breath movements during inhalation and exhalation. Perhaps you would like to direct your attention to the stream of air that flows through your nose into your lungs and back out again. If thoughts or memories should arise, allow them to pass by and direct your attention to your breath again. I would like to introduce you to a type of breathing in which we inhale and exhale for an equal length of time. When we do this, it helps to silently count. For example, we begin with 1...2...3...when you inhale and 1...2...3...when you exhale. Repeat this for another two to three times and notice how it feels. Perhaps this is the appropriate rhythm for you, or perhaps it's too fast. Then you can lengthen the phases and count 1...2...3...4...5...or more when you inhale and 1...2...3...4...5...or more when you exhale. I would like to once again emphasize that the goal is not to inhale and exhale as long as possible but make the inhalation and exhalation equally long.

Take time to sense what changes in your body when you control your breath. Perhaps you can do this exercise once again and check to see which speed feels best to you. You do not need to start with the gradual slowing of the breath each time but can start with the slow breathing right away, if this feels appropriate to you. If you are familiar with coherent breathing, you can also do it during the *asana* practice.

A female client gave me the following feedback: "When I practice coherent breathing, I inevitably start feeling stressed, because I think that I should manage this for longer. I'm always dissatisfied if I can just count to 3 or 4." We discussed this observation. It indicated one of the client's patterns that she was very familiar with. I suggested that she first try out some of the other *pranayama* exercises such as the Bee Breath, the Sun Breath, or *Ujjayi* Breath. These exercises automatically prolong the inhalation and exhalation. The client could also achieve her goal without having to fight for it.

After a while, it was possible to work with her beliefs of "I'm never good enough" and "I have to fight hard for everything." I initially wanted to create an experience of success for this client to contradict her old beliefs. Since practicing allowed her to feel that she received something without fighting for it, it was possible to "soften" her dysfunctional pattern a bit.

As already mentioned, we can also use physical exercises to send clients implicit therapeutic messages. In order to decide whether an exercise has advantages or whether we must offer something else to better pursue the therapeutic goals, we depend on feedback from clients.

SUN BREATH

In the Sun Breath we connect breath movements with rhythmic synchronous movements of the arms and hands. This *pranayama* practice automatically deepens the breath and helps clients to observe the breathing in a safer way since the focus is initially on the movement of the arms. The "distraction" helps many of them to feel relaxed despite the attention being placed on the breathing.

EXERCISE: SUN BREATH

If you like, try the following: Move your arms upward in front of your body as you inhale and downward as you exhale. How high you raise your arms and how quickly you do this movement is up to you... You can make very slow and gentle movements...or faster and more powerful...

Perhaps you would like to try out different variations to find out what is right for you at this moment.

You can also vary how high you would like to take your arms at any time... For example, up to shoulder height... You can also stretch them higher over your head...or...swing your arms up and down at the side instead of the front of the body...

We adapt the pattern to the person in front of us. We just suggest one or a maximum of two variations at one time. We can also speak about the interoceptive occurrence such as the weight of the arms, movement in the shoulder muscles, or changes in the chest or abdominal area. Some clients prefer to move the arms at the side instead of the front of the body. One client "invented" another variation by alternating the up and down movement of the arms as in walking, which allowed her to get into a swinging rhythm.

When practicing the Sun Breath, *prolonged exhalation* can be easily introduced.

EXERCISE: SUN BREATH WITH PROLONGED EXHALATION

If you like, you can stay with observing your breath rhythm for a moment... Perhaps the inhalation and exhalation are equally long...and perhaps there are differences...

Since the heartbeat slows down when you exhale and your nervous system calms down, I invite you to find out how it is to make the exhale a little longer than the inhale. As you do this, perhaps it will help you to count—while inhaling, slowly count to 3 or 4, and count to 4 or 5 or more when exhaling. The important thing is not to have any faltering of the breath or a sense of breathlessness. Only prolong the exhalation to the point where it feels quiet and pleasant.

UJJAYI BREATH—VICTORIOUS BREATH

Ujjayi (pronounced oo-jai) Breath can further intensify this slowing of the breath. How does the "Ocean Breath"—as it's also called—work?

EXERCISE: *UJJAYI* BREATH

Sit in a comfortable, upright posture. Inhale and exhale through the mouth a few times in a completely normal way... During the next exhale, imagine that you are breathing on a mirror. Now close your mouth and try the same thing again: You "breathe" on a mirror but keep your mouth closed as you do so... The next time that you inhale, maintain the constriction in your vocal cords... The sound may remind you of Darth Vader in the Star Wars films, whose breath sounded similar to this through his mask. Perhaps you would like to practice a few breaths with me in this form and observe what your body does... Perhaps you would like to focus on the area around your larynx and vocal cords...or perhaps feel the breath movements as such... You may sometimes also feel that your abdominal wall is rising and falling through the effort of breathing against the resistance... Or you notice something completely different.

Now I will take a break and let you practice a few breaths on your own in peace and quiet. You can stop at any time, no matter for what reason... So let's practice two or three more *Ujjayi* Breaths and then return to the normal breath rhythm.

The path of the air is practically extended since the same amount of air flows through less space. When we breathe through the nose, a mild contraction of the larynx muscles occurs, and a partial closing of the glottis occurs. Both of these elements increase the breath resistance and allow breath control. The clients automatically extend both the inhalation and the exhalation. This "sound of the sea" in the throat does not come from the vocal cords but is caused by the slight constriction of the throat. This way of breathing is said to stimulate the vagal afferent nerves, which leads to an activation of the parasympathetic nervous system.

PRACTICE TIP: For some clients, learning the *Ujjayi* Breath is a difficult endeavor. We can suggest variations with an open mouth to these clients and stay with it until this becomes easy. We can make the suggestion to try it with a closed mouth later.

Since *Ujjayi* Breath can dry out the vocal cords, it should not be practiced indefinitely. I also recommend that clients practice this type of breathing, as well as the Bee Breath, at home, so they can do something that is self-calming. As applies to all of our suggestions, the effect must obviously be examined in advance.

BHRAMERI BREATH—BEE BREATH

Like singing, the Bee Breath also automatically extends exhalation. In this exercise, make an even, deep, and powerful tone that sounds like the bee buzzing as you exhale. The exhalation can be supplemented by an additional effect if you cover your ears as you hum. Then you can feel the sound as a vibration in the head and chest area. This is where the acoustic effects connect with the kinesthetic experiences in which the hearing is coupled with a physical sensation.

EXERCISE: BEE BREATH

I invite you to make yourself comfortable and sit up as straight as possible to become familiar with the Bee Breath... Take a few relaxed inhales and exhales and make sure that your jaw and mouth are relaxed and your rows of teeth are not touching each other while your mouth is closed... Start by consciously inhaling through your nose and connect the exhalation with a humming tone... I'll demonstrate it for you...

Now try this out yourself and repeat it several times. If it feels pleasant to you, we can practice together for a few more moments. You can end the Bee Breath at any time.

Another possibility is covering your ears with both hands...and breathe in the same way. After a few more breaths, let your hands lower and observe the sensation of these sound vibrations for a moment.

ALTERNATING BREATH

Alternating Breath is understood as inhaling and exhaling through just one nostril. When the inhalation and exhalation is equally long, the effect is balancing. This means that the sympathetic nervous system and parasympathetic nervous system are balanced. Yoga says that the sun and moon energy, male and female, and the right and left side are harmonized. In the Alternating Breath, you can generate as many rhythms as you like by changing the inhale and/or exhale phases and take breaks in breathing.

EXERCISE: ALTERNATING BREATH

I invite you to try out the Alternating Breath with me. To do this, raise your right hand... Press your right thumb lightly against your right nasal wing to close the nostril... Now inhale through your left nostril... Fill your lungs about two-thirds of the way... Now close both nostrils with your thumb and index finger. Open the right nostril and exhale, during which you almost completely empty your lungs. Repeat this process a few times and stay attentive to what shows up in your body through this type of breathing.

Prolonged exhale: If you like, deliberately prolong the exhalation and create a new rhythm into the breathing... For example, count to 4 when you inhale and to 6 when you exhale...and stay connected with your experience... Also check what is appropriate for you. Try out which rhythm fits you at the moment... Perhaps you would like to inhale more deeply, perhaps exhale more, or perhaps return to an even rhythm.

Breath breaks: After the inhale, take a break and come up with a different rhythm. For example, count to 4 as you inhale, hold your breath as you count to 4 again, and finally exhale as you count up to 4. You can generate any rhythm in this way.

With training, it becomes increasingly easier for clients to prolong the exhalation and therefore activate the parasympathetic nervous system. If clients manage to pause their breath while inhaling, suggest that they take a break while exhaling. Here is a possible rhythm at the start: Inhale for 4, hold for 4, exhale for 4, hold for 4 (cf. Fuchs 2007).

Note that the nasal wings are just lightly closed, not pressed shut. This prevents the drying out of the nasal mucosa.

When we instruct yoga *asanas* and *pranayama*, we have our focus on various goals. We like to promote interoception, as well as experiencing in the here and now. Traumatic memories play out in the body and automatically draw attention away from the present to the past. We like to support clients in being able to tolerate and regulate arising thoughts, sensations, and emotions so that they have something in hand and no longer feel completely at the mercy of these traumatic memories.

BHASTRIKA BREATH—BELLOWS BREATH

In addition to a dynamic breathing rhythm that can be synchronized with powerful movements, Bellows Breath is another possibility for activating the sympathetic nervous system. Its special attribute is a quick consecutive forced inhale and exhale, like a blacksmith moving the bellows in a fast rhythm. Through this dynamic breathing, the belly is moved outward during the inhale and drawn back inward during the exhale. In this exercise, the lungs are expanded in a quick succession and contracted again, which produces a powerful hissing sound.

The starting posture is Mountain Pose (see Chapter 13) while seated. We inhale powerfully and audibly, and then push the air out in the same powerful and audible way. In *Bhastrika Breath*, a paradoxical breathing becomes clearly visible. If clients have become accustomed to this type of frightened breathing, they pull in their belly during the inhale and raise the chest. This gives us the possibility of exploring a different type of breathing together with the clients.

To generate a feeling for this powerful breathing, we first suggest three to four slow breaths at the start. Once clients have no difficulty (any more) with it, the speed can be increased. The Bellows Breath is practiced for a maximum of ten breaths, and then we always take a break. It can produce a mild feeling of dizziness, so we always start slow!

EXERCISE: BELLOWS BREATH

I invite you to try out a dynamic type of breathing. The best way is to start in Mountain Pose. Take your time and make sure that you are comfortable. I will show you how to do the Bellows Breath. During the strong inhalation and exhalation, move your belly actively like a bellows... When you inhale like this... [I demonstrate]...and when you exhale, you pull in your belly just as actively, like this... [I demonstrate].

This type of breathing is done with a maximum of ten breaths, which are always followed by a break. We start out slowly. When you are ready, inhale powerfully together with me...exactly...the belly curves outward...and now exhale powerfully...the belly moves inward...exactly like this... If this is appropriate for you, we will repeat it together in a rhythm that you determine.

Once clients are familiar with the *Bhastrika* Breath, the tempo can gradually be increased. It helps some clients to place their hands on their belly to experience the feeling of movement more intensively.

PRACTICE TIP: The Bellows Breath can trigger a sense of fear, so it can serve as exposure when the fear cannot be felt in the therapy setting. A careful approach and verbal support are important preconditions for clients having positive experiences. They can feel their fear through the breath, tolerate it, and learn to control it over time.

15

MINDFULNESS

As we have already discovered, all meditative traditions teach the value-free contemplation of the constantly changing inner and/or outer stimuli. When attention wanders away, clients return to the inner collection as soon as they become aware of this. The positive effects on the body and psyche have been repeatedly proven in many studies. Since the concept of *sati* or mindfulness tends to be foreign to the Western mind, the question arises as to which components are effective during the practice.

EFFECTIVE FACTORS

Bishop and his team (2004) suggest a two-component model. The first is the self-regulation of attention. For this purpose, clients focus their attention on the direct experience in the current moment, and observe the constantly changing thoughts, emotions, and physical sensations. This experience is frequently accompanied by the sense of being alert, present, and alive in the here and now. The second component is the inner attitude with which we encounter this experience. It is characterized by curiosity, openness, and acceptance—in which all of the experiences are equally accepted. This emphasizes the compassionate quality of mindfulness, which is characterized by a friendly interest in the present moment (cf. also Santorelli 1999).

Shapiro *et al.* (2006) supplement these two components of attention and inner attitude with an additional term: intention. From their point of view, intentional attention and non-judgmental openness lead to a significant change of perspective. This is described as "reperceiving." The better the meditators can detach themselves from the contents of consciousness, which means just observing them, the less they will get carried away by them. They experience the contents of consciousness

be getting a pillow because of an uncomfortable seat or creating a more appropriate distance. The clients notice that these actions have effects on their mental state. By developing the ability for relational mindfulness, they can connect the information that they have acquired through it with their inner mindfulness.

OBSERVING AND ACCOMPANYING MINDFULNESS

An "observing" mindfulness brings a distance between ourselves and what is happening; by contrast, an "accompanying" mindfulness allows us to stay closer to the experience.

In yoga, we establish an observer who monitors what is happening in a neutral and non-judgmental way. This distanced way of observing is not that simple, however, especially when traumatic events are involved. It's easier to assume a yoga position and observe a muscle contraction. This non-judging observation can be introduced and practiced bit by bit so that clients can increasingly allow themselves to be closer to the experience.

This distanced attitude of mindful observation is initially required to even develop an ability for affect regulation. When the ability for mindful observation grows, a mindful accompaniment also gradually begins. Whatever happens is allowed to come closer emotionally, and the individual history no longer needs to be kept at a distance. It can be processed and integrated. During this phase, emotions such as grief about what has been lost and missed out on, as well as anger about the injustice, desperation about the personal destiny, or empathy for the child who these people once were, also play an important role. This process begins when clients are able to observe emotions and physical sensations without being drawn into them or allowing themselves to be overwhelmed by them.

I frequently observe that it's hardly possible at first to experience grief about the personal destiny or empathy for the child who clients once were. Clients often resist the idea of the "inner child" and must fight off these painful and frequently shameful feelings for reasons that are quite understandable. The transition from the distanced, observing mindfulness to the closer, accompanying mindfulness is an important step. It can only be completed when clients have developed enough containment to tolerate their feelings.

BEING NON-JUDGMENTAL

As already mentioned, further aspects of mindfulness are acceptance and non-judgment. When not duly considered, these concepts can produce feelings of resignation. This happens when they are understood as accepting passive behavior—the simple acceptance of whatever happens to or is done with someone. That would be the opposite of what we want to offer our clients as new variants of action. "But I spent years putting up with him treating me like that. I am probably already very good at accepting!" This is the annoyed statement from a woman who had stayed with her violent husband for years when she was confronted with this concept in a book about mindfulness.

In turn, I consider acceptance and non-judgment from a "humanistic" perspective. By encouraging clients to observe what is happening in their body, we simultaneously encourage them to assume a curious-inquiring attitude. If this is too strenuous, they feel nothing at all or something different than what we have suggested—so nothing of this is assessed. Our own example can help clients in learning to notice their own sensations by observing without pigeonholing them.

So we encourage our clients to change something when it feels unpleasant or hurts. Or even trying out something different if they would like to. Unpleasant sensations should not simply be accepted and tolerated. They are an opportunity to make a decision and to take action.

For example, a mindful course of action is when clients notice that their foot hurts while in a pose. They can take the pressure off the foot by sitting up a bit straighter and noticing that the foot no longer hurts. At the same time, they sense less tension in the thigh muscles. When clients learn to mindfully observe this process, new "channels" can be created.

CASE EXAMPLE: BEING NON-JUDGMENTAL

A client (Mr. H) is in a very agitated state and notices that he can hardly breathe at that moment. I suggest a forward bend to him since this *asana* has a calming effect on him.

Mr. H: But isn't it wrong that I always do something about it when things get bad? Shouldn't I learn to tolerate it and stay with it?

DH: You can observe the arousal and also mindfully notice what happens when you decide to go into a forward bend.

Mr. H: Now it's better, but I feel bad because I wanted to tolerate it for longer.

DH: This is an interesting way of looking at it. For example, you could now observe how you feel better. And at the same time, you can explore what self-incriminations do in your body.

Mr. H: Hmmm... I never looked at it like that. The forward bend takes away some of the arousal, and I get more air again. The guilt feelings make my chest tighter again.

DH: And you can observe both again—the effect of the *asanas* and that of your thoughts.

Mr. H: By allowing both of them and staying in the pose, things get wider and lighter again in my chest.

At this point in time, I don't discuss the Mr. H's guilt feelings. I also do not try to influence the reassessment of his beliefs in a cognitive way; that would contradict the non-judgment. I lead him back to his body; nothing needs to be evaluated or changed. This simple observation affects a change.

WHAT DOES NON-MINDFULNESS ACTUALLY LOOK LIKE?

We are rarely attentive and completely in the here and now. If we leave the present in an unintentional way, our attention wanders to the past and we revel in memories or are overtaken by them. Or we move into the future. Then we make plans, struggle with fears and worries, or lose ourselves in reveries.

Mindfulness focuses more on the present. Sensory experiences receive a greater significance within this context, and these are precisely what interests us in yoga. We train them by facing the interoceptive occurrences. The best anchor for the present is the sensory experience.

CONCENTRATION AND MINDFULNESS EXERCISES

As we have already seen, all of the *asanas* and *pranayama* exercises are possibilities for practicing concentration and mindfulness. While I don't offer mindfulness exercises in silence to trauma clients, we can find a plethora of ideas for further "pure" mindfulness exercises in books by authors such as Kabat-Zinn (2007).

PART VI

ACHIEVING THERAPEUTIC GOALS WITH TRAUMA-SENSITIVE YOGA

As described at the start of this book, we are dealing with a variety of issues.

Therapeutic work with clients who suffer from complex trauma can be a minefield—we don't know where the mines are located or what triggers them. Even when we have initiated the upset and the client "winds up" in a state of dissociation or hyperarousal, we sometimes still do not know why. Since the speech center in the brain is not active in a state of arousal, clients can rarely articulate and explain what the trigger was. Such experiences do not lead to a trusting, viable therapeutic relationship. In this process, we are in danger of sidestepping to other less harmful topics that superficially serve to develop the relationship but that avoid work on the trauma and change nothing about the symptoms.

People with a complex trauma history torment themselves with a variety of symptoms and mental states. This can prevent them from taking charge of their life or make them unable to shape it according to their own ideas. This obviously includes the classic PTSD symptoms such as arousal, dissociation, sleep disorders, and nightmares, but also physical complaints such as chronic pain, anxiety and panic attacks, or difficulties on an interpersonal level—both in their professional and private life.

If we once again ask why these symptoms do not stop, we encounter rigid patterns of movement and posture that keep the stress in the system, and unbearable physical sensations that sustain the somatoform dissociation and alienation—in addition to frozen thought patterns. These phenomena prevent those affected from establishing connections with other people. On the one hand, they avoid closer contacts or live dysfunctional relationship patterns due to their traumatic experiences; on the other hand, they often have difficulty in a natural and carefree interaction with others.

For the therapeutic relationship, this means that in order to develop a stable relationship, these clients require tools to help them to regulate their affects and to deal with their internal and external triggers as a result. At the same time, the relationship must be shaped in such a way that the affected individuals feel secure and their experience is as different as possible from the experience of the trauma. This part of the book discusses how we can encounter the above-mentioned hurdles with specific yoga interventions.

16

OVERVIEW OF THERAPY GOALS AND TRAUMA-SENSITIVE YOGA

The following table shows the different impacts of trauma. It's obvious that complex traumas and even more developmental traumas lead to much more complex symptoms. It is, as mentioned above, not always clear that the variety of symptoms have their cause in traumas like abuse or neglect. Patients often come to therapy because they cannot deal properly with their life, work situation or relationships, and don't feel like a "trauma survivor." We have to make the link between symptoms and causes.

Symptoms	Therapeutic goal	Trauma-Sensitive Yoga interventions
Pull of the past through dissociation and flashbacks	Affect regulation, here-and-now experiencing	Orientation in the present through mindfulness training, interoceptive perception, and influencing the nervous system through breath
Constant inner and muscular tension	Relaxation	Rhythmic instruction—observing the sensations of tension and relaxation in the musculature, short breaks of silent noticing of sensations
Numbing—the feeling that nothing is changing Atony	Perception of changes	Breaks—observation of changes after *asanas* or *pranayama* Activating, dynamic, and powerful *asanas*
Dissociation	Orientation in the here and now	Powerful *asanas* and breathing
Sympathetic—activating rapid breathing	Subduing of a sympathetic nervous system reaction Activation of a relaxation reaction	Perceiving breath as movement, slowing breath, extending exhale, breathing with "sound," such as Bee Breath or *Ujjayi* Breath
Parasympathetic—activating shallow breathing	Interrupting of the shut-down reaction Activating of sympathetic nervous system	Deepening breath, breath synchronized with dynamic movements
Holding the breath		Reminder to breathe
Relationship traumatization—"The other person is the trigger"	Developing therapeutic relationship, trust, and sense of security	Mirroring, staying in contact with the voice, no judging or assessing; practicing, learning, and exploring together
Rejection of own body, shame, and disgust	Building resources	Finding body areas with positive or neutral connotations; functional language

Feeling of alienation from own body	Sensing the body again	Interoceptive training, exposure, allowing time—non-myelinated nerve fibers require time
Avoidance of physical sensations/triggers in the body	Learning to tolerate physical sensations	Gentle exposure training through interoceptive exploration and habituation
Overwhelmed by physical reactions and feelings; hyperarousal	Affect regulation, learning to "step on the brakes"; control	Calming *pranayama* exercises and *asanas*—learning to influence the nervous system
Concentration problems	Improve concentration	Concentration and mindfulness exercises, interoceptive awareness
Frozen postures and inflexible movement patterns that cement the traumatic state into the body	Flexibility in posture and movement	Dynamic *asanas*; perceiving movement when assuming and releasing a pose; perceiving movement; perceiving breathing as movement
Incomplete movements and defensive strategies	Having defensive strategies available again	Perceiving movement; getting moving; deciding on movement; feeling impulses and giving in to them
Relationship as a trigger	Avoiding the ventral vagus	Relaxed voice and facial expressions when accompanying and instruction, being in a state of relaxation
Asymmetrical relationship pattern	Relationship on an equal basis	No evaluating or judging—no attitude of "expertise"
Loss of control and helplessness	Empowerment	Control over the type of performance, duration, choices, and open and inviting formulations
Feelings of inferiority; fears of failure	Self-esteem	Choice and variations of exercises means that there are no errors and therefore no failure

17

PSYCHOEDUCATION

If we want to make people do something they are afraid of and have therefore more or less successfully avoided, we need good reasons. These include background information on the origin of the trauma and the hypotheses for trauma healing, including treatment possibilities. Depending on the therapeutic procedures with which we work, trauma therapists develop their personal use of language with which to convince clients to participate in trauma therapy and exposure. This is why I focus only on body therapy aspects here since they can flow into every type of trauma therapy at this point.

In addition to the various other clinical questionnaires already mentioned, I use the questionnaire by Nijenhuis on Somatoform Dissociation (SDQ-5 or SDQ-20) when making a diagnosis (Nijehuis *et al.* 1996). This allows me to focus the client's attention on the relationship between trauma and the body, which facilitates a conversation about the meaningfulness of including the body in the therapy.

In the initial phase, I use a sketch to explain how the cascade of defense (see Chapter 3) works. This serves to clarify that this process occurs time and again in their everyday life when triggers appear. In addition to emotional reactions, I also emphasize the physical aspects for this purpose. These include body postures and breathing, as well as physical sensations such as a lump in the throat, palpitations, pressure in the stomach area, rigidity—sensations that could be linked with anger, fear, and the feelings of powerlessness and helplessness. Understanding how these survival mechanisms run reflexively—which means that they cannot be controlled by thinking and the rational mind—is a relief to many clients. "So it isn't my fault that I react like this?" is a frequent reaction to this explanation.

Sometimes I make another sketch to illustrate the development of a fear network (see Chapter 18) as a consequence of traumatization. If I already have information about it, I use the triggers that were previously recognized by the client and emphasize specific physical sensations that could become triggers here. This gives me the opportunity to make the role of avoidance—both the outer and somatic inner triggers—comprehensible. Furthermore, we speak about numbness and the sense of being cut off from the body, as well as dissociation, as a protective measure for survival.

Now I can explain in understandable terms why we slow down these unconscious, fast-moving processes, and initially have to develop braking strategies as resources that clients can use when the pull of the memories gets the upper hand. In order to gain these resources, we do not work with excessive arousal. We never tackle the traumas during the first hours. Instead, we work with clients to test what helps them to stay in the here and now and to calm themselves again. I often get the feedback that these explanations have a very calming effect, since the client no longer needs to fear that they will automatically experience the same things in the therapy as in everyday life—being overwhelmed by memories and feelings that they cannot tolerate. Of course, we cannot guarantee with absolute certainty that this will not happen, since we must first get to know the clients.

In the last step I explain how the practical approach will look, that we will systematically work during the first hours of therapy to find simple body postures and also breathing exercises from yoga that will give clients a greater sense of security and calmness. In the following therapy sessions we try to solidify these, so that clients can use them in everyday life when the memories threaten to overwhelm them. Since yoga offers very clear and structured exercises, it is well suited as a precaution against losing control, helplessness, and powerlessness.

The next chapter contains case examples that substantiate this practical approach.

18

PRACTICE AND CASE EXAMPLES

BUILDING RESOURCES

When clients are incapable of feeling their body because it just reacts with being overwhelmed or dissociation, or when they are disgusted at themselves, ashamed of their body, feel dirty, etc., the body can't be used for affect regulation. This is why we look for somatic resources at the beginning of our work in TSY. We first try to help clients direct their attention to neutral or pleasant body zones or parts of the body. This can only work when the arousal isn't too strong because the pull of overwhelming memories and therefore emotions and sensations is too vehement. The idea of starting with yoga means that initially we do not do "exposure therapy" in the actual sense of the word; instead, we set off in search of resources by approaching the body and its sensations with various *asanas* and *pranayama*.

I tend to start the yoga sequences with seated Mountain Pose (see Chapter 13). This is a basic posture that we can always return to. If this pose is a trigger that reminds clients of previous traumatic experiences, I select a different *asana*. For example, this could be Staff Pose, standing Mountain Pose, or even an entirely individual pose—it doesn't have to be a "textbook" *asana*.

After we have taken our places on the "yoga chairs" or chosen a place to stand, I invite clients to make themselves comfortable in the space, to choose the right spot to stand or sit, perhaps correct the distance between them and me, or to check to see whether they would rather have their back to the wall instead of the window. When they have found a good place, we start by assuming the first *asana* and directing the focus to the feet, for example. How to assume this pose, as well as variations of Mountain Pose and other *asanas*, is described in Chapter 13.

The dialog in the phase of finding resources could look something like this:

> When you are ready, try to direct your attention to your feet... Perhaps first sense your contact with the floor...by moving your feet and toes a bit... And while you do this, ask yourself whether contact with your feet is possible...and how you perceive it. For example, through the temperature, texture, or something entirely different...

We may be able to ask how being in touch with the floor with their feet makes them feel—whether this has a positive, neutral, or negative effect on their mental state. So I invite clients to notice any sensations or to check to see whether this tends to cause good or negative feelings or unpleasant physical reactions within them.

If contact of the feet with the floor leads to a positive sensation, which means that activation of the nervous system is reduced, we stay with exploring resources so that they become anchored in the client's consciousness.

But if contact with the feet triggers negative sensations and feelings that increase the activation of the nervous system, we go on a joint search for a remedy. When clients exhibit clear signs of stress in the form of dissociation and freezing, I check with them to see whether a change of focus to a different body area with neutral or positive connotations, a different posture, or physical movement may become a resource and contribute to their relief, for example, doing shoulder rolls...or Cat–Cow movements. A further possibility is a change of perspective through a Spinal Twist, Downward Dog Pose, or a standing pose. For some clients, immobility can also be resolved through powerful movements. In the same sense, the feeling of muscle power and strength—such as in a Warrior Pose, Chair Position, or Staff Pose—can also become a resource when clients tend to dissociate.

Once a helpful posture has been found, I invite clients to stay in it but to remain in verbal contact so that this pausing doesn't transform into rigidity and immobility. I address the interoceptive sensations, remind them of the flow and movement of the breath, and talk about the possibility of changing something at any time. For example, counting the breaths helps clients to comprehend that the overwhelming emotions and sensations won't continue endlessly.

The following example from practice, which is an excerpt from my first session with the client, illustrates this creative search for resources.

CASE EXAMPLE: LISA

Lisa is a 34-year-old woman who was sexually abused by a male relative for years during her childhood. We talk about her first childhood memories, and I see how she stiffens and contracts. I suggest tracking down the physical expression of these memories.

Lisa: Everything inside of me gets tense, and I make myself small. Sometimes I stamp my feet really hard on the floor so that I can still feel that I'm "here" and tense up even more...

She has clenched her hands into fists. Her shoulders are drawn forward and tense. I initially don't mention her feet but focus attention on her hands.

DH: Perhaps you would like to start by directing your attention to your fingers...

Lisa: They are tense.

She squeezes them even tighter together, and her knuckles are completely white.

DH: And perhaps you can take a look at your hands...and try to gradually let go of your fingers and open your hands... just that...

Lisa slowly opens her fists.

Lisa: My arms are also a bit more relaxed now...

DH: And would you like to try to open your shoulders a bit at a time...

Lisa moves her shoulders back, together with her arms. She opens them widely and tilts her head back.

DH: Do you perhaps sense your chest muscles or arms during this movement...?

Lisa: I can really feel the muscles in my neck... This is unpleasant...and it doesn't feel good to tilt my head so far back...

DH: Try to open your chest again while looking straight ahead or continue to look down...

Lisa follows my suggestion.

Lisa: Holding my head high means being self-confident, and that's not what I am...

DH: When I lower my head, I notice that I perceive very little from the outside... And perhaps it's also good for you to be able to see just a little of the outside now...

Lisa: I can't tolerate any more right now... I just see my legs and feet...that's enough! What I notice is that I'm pressing my feet into the floor and my legs are getting tense...

DH: Perhaps you would like to try coming into Staff Pose... [I demonstrate.] This means stretching out your legs... and pulling up your toes...and then relaxing again...Lisa follows me and tries out the movements.

Lisa: Pulling up my toes isn't good since it creates more tension...stretching is better...

DH: Then leave your toes and feet totally relaxed or stretch them out...and see how this is...

She tries out both and chooses stretching.

Lisa: This is better...

DH: I notice that I clearly feel my sit bones in Staff Pose... My entire weight is resting on them...

Lisa: Yes, I also sense this, and it feels good... It's more pleasant than feeling the weight on my feet...

She stays in this posture for a moment, then takes her hands away from her lap and lets them hang down. I do the same.

DH: Now there is even more weight on the sit bones...

Lisa: Yes, and now I feel totally calm and relaxed...

We stay in this posture for a moment and then release it together.

At the beginning of the therapy I consciously avoid sensations that have a "negative" connotation. This means that I do not explore how clients perceive contact with the floor if it triggers stress. This is why I initially spend time on the hands and only later on the feet, for example.

One of my male clients said: "But isn't that also avoidance?" He was obviously right, but as long as clients do not yet feel adequately secure in "putting on the brakes," I quite consciously want to avoid an intensive sympathetic activation and also a parasympathetic nervous system shut-down. Depending on the physical experiences during the traumatization, entire body regions such as the buttocks, genitals, chest, or legs can be "not okay" and initially not serve as a resource. "Not okay" can also mean that these body regions are taboo in the eyes of the affected person because they are "ugly." This is where a functional language helps us to speak about muscles, joints, stretching, activity, weight, etc.

Finding resources requires us to be creative. As mentioned above, even just the movements—the feeling of being able to move—can represent an important resource. *Asanas* that imply movement such as the Sun Breath or Cat–Cow allow the affected person to sense that they are capable of moving their bodies, and this is often perceived as empowerment. The muscle activity that clients experience in Warrior Pose or Chair Position can give them confidence and trust in their own strength or remind them of their power. People who feel themselves to a very minor degree or hardly at all can get adequate stimuli through looking, moving, touching textures, or sensing temperature differences to determine how something feels in their body. They could touch muscles that are active at that moment in the pose, for example, feeling their abdominal muscles with their hands when leaning back. I have often received feedback that it helps to see me do a movement so that it can be perceived in the client's body.

Working out resources is one of the most important elements of trauma therapy. Without resources, we are unable to help clients to counteract their past experiences. No matter whether assuming, holding, or releasing the *asanas* or *pranayama*, the key is interoception. Being able to feel the body in a neutral way at the very least is a major and important step for healing.

AFFECT REGULATION AND CONTROL

If clients have some somatic resources and increased body awareness, we can start with the next step, which is to teach clients how to slow down sympathetic arousal and/or prevent the shut-down of their dorsovagal parasympathetic nervous system. This is how they can expand their personal window of tolerance. Learning doesn't take place when the client is overwhelmed of emotions or dissociated, because he is no longer within his personal/individual window of tolerance. Being able to control his affects means he is within the window of tolerance and only in this controlled state does learning take place.

While there are various possibilities for toning down an arousal, the leitmotif is focusing on something that triggers a ventrovagal parasympathetic activity. This can be achieved with positive images such as photos on a mobile phone or a family photo in a wallet. But it is also possible through visualizing a safe place (Reddemann 2001). Acoustic signals—a female client had saved the voice of a girlfriend on her mobile phone, which got her back into the here and now when she had a flashback—are another possibility, and somatic resources are obviously also included.

A resource must be available and memorable when the client's stress level is high. Although visualizations fulfill this criterion, creating an inner image is an act that leads away from the body and therefore away from interoceptive awareness. This requires access to cognitive abilities, which tend to be blocked by a strong affect. In contrast to the visualization, the feeling of a physical sensation is controlled by the subcortical regions of the brain.

A female client said this, with a wink: "That's good. I always have my body with me!"

One first, important step here is that clients learn to deliberately direct their attention away from the sensations that reanimate the traumatic occurrence and to focus on other somatic stimuli. Doing so requires adequately strong, distinct stimuli that allow them to hold this focus.

However, there is a good reason why clients do not want to direct the focus to their body at the first sign of an arousal. They ultimately fear nothing more than feeling that they are at the helpless mercy of their somatic sensations. The fear of these uncontrollable waves is significant. In this case, they feel that it's safer to split off from their bodies. Quite a few of my clients already dissociate at the suggestion of focusing on the body. Quiet sitting thwarts this concern of developing more body awareness since we can hardly feel our shoes on our feet or our clothing on our skin after sitting in a chair or armchair for a while.

This interoceptive awareness only succeeds—as already mentioned—through change in position.

Let's return to the yoga practice. By focusing our attention on an active muscle, the holding of one hand, or the position of a foot, or the movement and flow of the breath, we concentrate on it. When we change to a different *asana*, the change of posture results in new stimuli and therefore new focus possibilities. Yoga is a constant practicing of narrowing our focus and concentrating (*dharana*, an important step in the Eightfold Path).

How does slowing down work in TSY? Overwhelming sensations and emotions come fast and uncontrollable, and clients are not able to control or slow them down to make the experience more bearable. Slowing down the process allows the client to get more control instead of helplessness. An example from practice explains this approach.

CASE EXAMPLE: SANDRA

Here I describe one phase from a session at the start of the therapy process. I very much strove at this point in time to have Sandra perceive and slow down the little activations. The interoceptive perception and resource situation had not yet been expanded to the extent that we could deal with the stronger arousals.

We do not sit directly across from each other so that her eyes can look into the distance when they are open. I also do the same thing when Sandra keeps her eyes closed. We start with seated Mountain Pose.

Sandra tries out the various movements and positions. She finds a good place for her feet. She keeps her eyes closed and nods. She seems relaxed. Her breath is calm.

DH: You can leave your eyes closed but also open them at any time. Sometimes it's more pleasant to have your eyes closed, and sometimes contact with the outside is important to orient yourself. [We have spoken about how orientation in space can have a calming effect because this lets her once again "know" where she is.]

She nods and keeps her eyes closed.

Sandra: Sensing my feet feels good to me once again. It gives me support.

DH: That's good, and you can return back to your feet and the support at any time... Whatever I suggest, please consider it and decide whether it feels right to you... You can change something about it at any time... Go ahead and stay with your feet for another moment...and then sit up a bit straighter when it's okay for you...

Sandra sits up straight and moves her shoulders.

DH: Exactly... You can also use your shoulders to help you... and feel which role they play when you sit up straight...

Since Sandra has her eyes closed, I comment on her movements, so that she senses she has my attention. I also do the shoulder movements, regardless of her closed eyes.

Sandra: Yes, I know... I am familiar with sitting up straight from my physiotherapy...the string at the crown that pulls me up higher.

DH: Yes, you can do it like that if this idea is helpful...or you can also sense how your body would like to sit up straight at this moment...

Sandra keeps trying, finds a pleasant upright position, and opens her eyes. She sits a bit lopsided on the chair.

Sandra: I'm not as upright as I thought I was, and not as stiff.

DH: Exactly. This is how sitting up straight feels to YOU TODAY (I emphasized the "you" and "today")... And perhaps you want to explore how to straighten up somewhat more intensively by making little or bigger movements back and forth.

Sandra closes her eyes again, starts to rock slightly, and takes a deep breath.

DH: And if it feels right to you, you can also try movements from one side to the other.

Sandra also tries out this movement pattern.

Sandra: This is nice...

DH: If you want, you can also connect the movements and make circles...

Sandra nods. But instead of doing the circling movements, she stiffens. I suggest that she opens her eyes and notices whether that makes a difference. She nods and confirms my assumption that opening her eyes somewhat diminishes the arousal. I ask her what has just changed within her body.

Sandra: When I imagine it, the circling doesn't feel good to me. I feel pressure on my chest.

DH: It's good that you noticed this... Now try to return your attention to your feet... Perhaps you can also look down at your feet on the floor...

Sandra looks down, then straight ahead again, and takes a deep breath.

Sandra: Better!

DH: Good...stay with your feet as long as it feels good to you.

Sandra: Now it's good again.

She takes a deep breath and her body tension has visibly relaxed.

Something had triggered Sandra—possibly the circling movements or that she had had enough interoceptive exploration of her body center for now. It was important that she noticed how she got the proverbial ground beneath her feet when she directed her attention at them.

At the beginning of the therapy, I rely completely on avoidance until enough regulation ability has been developed. This means that I help clients release their attention from an unpleasant sensation and search for and focus on a neutral or positive sensory perception instead. Is this case, we can go one step further and alternate between a somatic resource and a somatic trigger.

We guide clients in going back and forth between a positive or neutral and an unpleasant physical sensation, and direct their attention from one physical sensation to the other. The alternating helps clients to better tolerate sensations and emotions.

In many cases, this is a helpful method to slow down this process. The redeeming anchor must become established and practiced in a lower state of arousal. This allows it to become something familiar that is really available to clients "in case of an emergency."

This alternating is often not that simple, however, because the pull of the trauma is essentially much stronger than the trust in a resource. However, I have had the experience that it becomes easier when this process is connected to a concrete action such as changing posture/ perspective or activating the muscles.

A few sessions later, Sandra was more familiar with her somatic resources and had had good experiences with getting a grip on the little arousals once again. This is why we began working with a "higher charge." We started with setting up seated Mountain Pose, with which she was already familiar, and she felt that the contact of her feet with the floor was pleasant. As a new element, I suggested that she concentrate on the movement of her breath.

Sandra: Breath is a word that immediately frightens me.

She opens her eyes and looks around.

DH: Where do you feel the fear?

Sandra: It's always there.

She points to her chest and slumps a bit. I ask her to notice this and then once again concentrate on her feet as in Mountain Pose and moving them, etc.

Sandra: This is so bad here. My feet are powerless there... I can't feel them anymore...

DH: Perhaps it helps to direct your eyes to your feet...see the movement...

Sandra looks down, moving her feet and toes.

DH: Exactly...and also move your toes...

I observe how she strokes her hands over her thighs.

DH: And perhaps now you feel your hands in addition to your feet...the contact...the warmth... Perhaps also take a look...

Sandra: Better...not great but better... Sensing my hands feels good.

She continually strokes her hands over her thighs.

DH: And feel free to stay a bit longer in contact with your hands and the movement of your hands... You may feel the fabric of your pants...the warmth beneath your hands...and perhaps also slowly come back into Mountain Pose...by sitting up a bit straighter...

The word, as well as the posture itself, serves as an anchor. Only mentioning a term like "seated Mountain Pose," which is linked with a good experience, can start a relaxation or calm the client. There is a difference between whether we should sit up and have a straight backbone or whether we should strive to assume a certain *asana*. The structure of the *asanas* helps to approach the form without the focus on "sit straight" triggering negative emotions. In addition, this one term involves a complex sequence of movements that clients can easily understand because they have practiced them.

Sandra relaxes, sits up a bit straighter, moves her shoulders, and breathes more deeply.

DH: ...And stay in Mountain Pose for a bit longer...

Sandra breathes a bit deeper again, and her hands are relaxed. After a few breaths, I venture a new attempt.

DH: ...Now it may be possible for you to once again make contact with the feeling in your chest of briefly being there... and then return your attention to your feet and hands, in Mountain Pose...

Sandra: This is difficult, but it's working a little better than before... It's better with my hands together...

We go back and forth several times between the sensations in the following minutes—it becomes increasingly easier for Sandra to focus on her chest.

Since many trauma-related triggers are located in the body and it becomes a dangerous or unreliable place, it's even more important to establish the opposite poles there. Clients often have a subconscious map of their body. Dark colours often indicate difficult zones (dirty, painful, fat, hurt, abused…). Working with the body can change this perception and dark colors can change into brighter colors. Or previously white zones, due to the lack of sensations, transform timidly into friendly, light color accents. For some clients, the idea of a body map is very attractive, so we design such a map together. For both clients and therapists, this is an equally good benchmark that shows how body awareness changes.

Another remedy for affect regulation is supporting clients in learning to differentiate between feelings, thoughts, and sensations.

LEARNING TO DIFFERENTIATE

In a state of intense arousal, feelings, sensations, and thoughts merge into a complex structure. If we succeed in separating and differentiating them, they no longer besiege the affected person with their entire force. Each individual element becomes somewhat more manageable as a result. The various components are often located in different ways within the body, but clients are unable to cope with them in the vortex of feelings and memories.

As one female client said:

> When we were children, we got little sticks of Play-Doh in six colors, nicely organized in a small carton. We shaped all kinds of things out of them. What we no longer liked, we kneaded into a lump and made something new out of it. So our Play-Doh changed over time into a gray mass that had colorful streaks running through it. Although the original colors could still be guessed, it was impossible to get them back out again.

This is exactly what our work is about. We "retrieve" the single components out of the gray, undifferentiated complex so that clients learn to deal with these individual elements.

An effective means of learning differentiation is the labeling that I became familiar with in mediation practice. Thoughts, feelings, memories, dreams, etc., arise during mediation. As soon as we become aware of them, we give them a label that can be general or more differentiated: "thoughts," "thinking," or "plan for the future," "feeling" or "grief," "anger," "physical sensation" or "pressure," or "pain." This labeling is usually done mentally instead of being spoken out loud, but we can always adapt it to the client's needs. After the labeling, we return our attention to the focus of mediation such as the breath.

This differentiating begins with the mindful observation of what is happening in the body. One muscle is stretched, but another is tensed. One side has space, but the other is a bit compressed. Clients gradually succeed in recognizing and naming the correlations between thoughts and physical sensations or between feelings and physical sensations. Here is an excerpt from another session with Sandra.

CASE EXAMPLE: SANDRA

We sit on the "yoga chairs"—which are staggered as we face each other, as Sandra had requested. We speak about the various occurrences during the past week. When a distressing memory arises, her previously straight back curves slightly. I draw her attention to this.

Sandra: I'm being pulled back down again.

We had already done the Cat–Cow movement, a forward bend, which is followed by a backbend, and practice the forward bend by itself. This is why I risk inviting her to follow this movement impulse. I consciously call the pose a "forward bend." Since Sandra was already familiar with this *asana*, this position had a functional yoga aspect in addition to the impulse of hunching over.

Sandra: That's like a pull! There's no more control when I go in there. Just fear.

DH: Exactly, you feel the pull...and you can slowly start sitting up straight again...as in the Cat–Cow...

I mirror her posture and start to very gently straighten up. Sandra stays where she is for a moment and then moves her upper body a bit vertically.

Sandra: Now I sense nothing but grief and a deserted space.

DH: We are dealing with two different things here. With the pull of the fear that paralyzes you...as well as with the desert and the grief... I presume that you are more present again when you are sad...

[Grief is not connected with the fight–flight–freeze reactions. As a result, clients come back more into the here and now again when they feel grief and pain. I had already discussed this with Sandra.]

Sandra: I had always thrown this into one pot... I hadn't even noticed that these are two entirely different feelings...

She seems relieved.

DH: Hmmm...this is good... Both of them together are a concentrated charge, but each on their own is easier to tolerate...

Sandra: Yes, now that I can differentiate between the two, not everything that I feel is "fear"...? I thought that everything was fear... It helps me greatly that I now have two pictures of two different things in my head.

DH: It's good when we can give the things a name and know what we are dealing with.

At the moment in which we put the right label on the feeling and can tell the feelings apart from each other, the cognitive part of the brain is active. We start to understand, and this means that we can integrate something on a cognitive level. Feelings are often linked with various body positions. For Sandra, the differentiation between somatic sensations and body postures makes an essential contribution to her ability to differentiate her feelings.

FLEXIBILITY IN POSTURE AND MOVEMENT

A trauma becomes visible in patterns of movement and posture. It does not matter whether the powerlessness and helplessness or a counterprogram, such as "I'll never be a victim again!," have become entrenched in the corporeality and behavior. Both lack the flexibility of assuming postures that allow people to experience the entire spectrum of the emotional world. Pat Ogden and colleagues write: "Chronic postural and movement tendencies serve to sustain certain beliefs and cognitive distortions, and the physical patterns, in turn, contribute to the maintenance of these same beliefs" (Ogden *et al.* 2006, p.47).

Subtle adaptations of the movement patterns to our social environment are always also expressed in body postures. When children are encouraged to live out their urge to move, they will move differently from those who are punished for this and garner disapproval. The continual repetition of certain movement patterns forms our psyche and our body. It influences our bodily functions. Children who already make themselves smaller at the sound of their father's key in the lock, hold their breath, and tense every muscle will automatically develop postural and movement patterns over time. There's a great probability that they will later experience pain in their shoulders and back.

In such a case, we can offer clients a gentle backbend to counter their accustomed body pattern since this will open up their chest, or a movement in the shoulders that loosens this chronically tensed area. It is a good idea to stay in this posture for a moment, as yoga intends. Then the experiences that arise can be explored. Sometimes even just an inch of movement can trigger a reaction, which is why a cautious approach is an absolute basic prerequisite within this context. The reactions to postures can also change during this work, and this is why I never think of myself as being in a safe area, even if I am offering something familiar. I am aware that I can set off a trigger with every suggestion.

The attitude of "not knowing," coupled with the focus on the here and now, is an advantage. If we remain in the past—in the last session—we leave too little space for the possibilities of change. Formulations such as "...how it feels today/now..." can help clients to gain such insights. For example, they may realize that things can change without us having to explicitly speak about restricting cognitions, such as "nothing will ever change."

If a body posture such as a backbend triggers a negative sensation and emotion, we have various possibilities. We could make suggestions and give clients ideas about how they can change the *asana* so that it becomes tolerable for them. We could also remind them that they can release the *asana* at any time. At a later time, we could risk a new attempt to approach the backbend by linking the *asana* with movement, for example. We could look at whether the difficulty is because clients hold their breath, and then suggest resuming the flow of the breath again. Afterward, when the arousal is within a tolerable scope, we could invite them to observe their breath movements and other interoceptively perceptible sensations. As described in the last section, we could also direct the focus to resources we have already worked out together. Or, if clients are able to cope, we can rock to and fro with them to slow down the arousal in this way.

CASE EXAMPLE: SANDRA

In a later session with Sandra, I introduced movement in the form of the Sun Breath after we set up Mountain Pose. Since breath was a problem for her, both as a concept and as a sensation, I combined breath and movement so that we didn't constantly avoid this topic. I hoped that this combination was tolerable for her.

DH: I suggest that we experiment today with breath and movement... So just try to see how it is if you raise your arms at your sides while inhaling...and lower them again while exhaling... You decide how high you would like to take your arms...and you determine the rhythm. Keep your eyes open or closed—however you like...

I knew that I was taking a "risk" by focusing on the breath again. At the same time, I saw this as an opportunity since Sandra primarily concentrated on her arms and not just her chest during the Sun Breath. She begins with the movements and I join her. Sandra starts out with timid movements, which I mirror. These movements slowly become bigger and more secure, and I adapt once again.

Sandra: This reminds me of flying.

She makes slow, even movements and her breath flows quietly and steadily.

DH: Yes, that's right... I've never seen it like that. We can perhaps stay with this movement for a few more breaths.... You may also feel how the muscles in your shoulders and upper back are working.

The focus on the muscles brings her attention to her body. Sandra clearly feels the contrast to the rigidity that arose with her fear.

Sandra lets her arms lower and puts her hands back on her thighs. She keeps her eyes closed.

DH: You can allow yourself a brief moment to take a break and notice any sensations.

Sandra: Wanting and allowing are such words! I can't handle them at all. My panic immediately increases. My chest gets tight.

I knew that I was provoking an arousal with these words—she had given me this feedback during the previous session. The physical reaction is immediately visible—her back hunches. She makes herself very small and her body stiffens. Her knees move inward, as do the tips of her toes. Her entire body stiffens.

Sandra: It's back again now—the fear.

DH: Perhaps you can direct your attention to your feet and notice that they are standing differently than usual on the floor... And you can try to move your feet in such a way that their tips point straight ahead.

She moves her feet a bit to the outside. Her knees follow.

DH: And perhaps it is now possible for you to straighten up a little in Mountain Pose so that your feet are once again giving you solid support.

I am now also in a forward bend and slowly start to straighten up in the same rhythm as Sandra. She is now sitting up straighter again. I suggest moving the shoulders up and down a bit.

Sandra: This feels good. I'm getting some air again.

Sandra opens her rib cage and visibly relaxes.

DH: And slowly allow the movements in the shoulder to get bigger... Perhaps also include your arms... and transition into a Sun Breath... Synchronize the movement with the breath, if you like... Bring your arms up while inhaling and move your arms back down while exhaling.

She nods, and we begin with the Sun Breath. After some movements and breaths:

DH: You can lift your arms up to shoulder height or try out how it is to move your arms entirely above your head.

Sandra stretches her arms in the direction of the ceiling and remains in this position.

Sandra: Stretching feels good.

But she simultaneously holds her breath and becomes increasingly stiff. I don't explicitly talk about my observations but make a suggestion to bring her out of this freeze.

DH: From this posture, you can do a side bend... I'll demonstrate it...and combine this in turn with your breath and movement by switching from right to left and back again... You also set the tempo here...and whether you would like to synchronize the movement with your breath.

Sandra leans to the right and then starts moving in a smooth motion. She has her eyes closed and visibly relaxes. Now that the arousal has settled, I once again risk talking about the breath and make her aware of her ribs and intercostal muscles. In a side bend, one side is stretched and the other shortened. This movement leads to an especially good perception of this muscle group during inhalation.

Sandra: Now I understand!

She stops in the middle of the movement and abruptly opens her eyes.

Sandra: The breath isn't the problem at all. When I inhale here, it doesn't do anything. It's this point here in my chest that contracts when the panic comes up.

All postures, movements and breathing exercises have to be done consciously, since sensorimotor perception requires time. The interoceptive neural pathways consist of small, slow A delta and C fibers that are non-myelinated and therefore slow-moving (Fogel 2009). Staying and exploring has a great value: "The ability of abstract logical thinking is so efficient and quick in human beings that it can impede the growth of embodied self-perception. Embodied self-perception required the slowing of our abstract mind so that it can recuperate from its continuous stream of assessment and time planning" (Fogel 2009, p.43).

IMPULSES AND INTERRUPTED DEFENSIVE MOVEMENT

Trauma can be understood as both a frozen posture and an interrupted defensive movement. Like breath, these movements occur involuntarily and voluntarily, as well as consciously and unconsciously. Our adaptive fixed-action patterns for defense consist of a multitude of movements that are carried out automatically. If a danger appears, our body reacts to it without any thought on our part. We experience anger or fear, the only purpose of which is to set us in motion. In the case of a traumatic experience, these emotions are very strong. They want to help us in fleeing or cause us to defend ourselves. If neither of these succeeds, we stay stuck in the movement and also in our emotions. Consequently, the same messages about incomplete movements and/ or action patterns arrive in the brain time and again. These unfinished defensive actions—which can arise as sensorimotor fragments in the form of body memories or movement impulses—often show up later as symptoms such as chronic tensed muscles or weakness in a certain region of the body. The emotional reactions are either exaggeratedly aggressive or inappropriately passive and defensive.

A treatment that helps people to overcome their trauma should also somehow take these facts into consideration. This means that we must design this therapy setting in such a way that impulses for movement and actions come to light so that we can work with them. This can allow the affected person to complete the interrupted defensive strategies.

Involuntary movements that clients show during a therapy session can indicate uncompleted action patterns—a defensive hand movement, an upper body that leans forward, feet that make little (walking) movements, etc. When we suggest that clients notice this movement and give space to the impulse, this can mean a major discharge and liberation.

Levine (2010) described discharges in animals as trembling, vibrating, shaking off, etc. In human beings, this can also be expressed in the form of relieving tears, hot flashes, or shivers. An omnipresent helplessness that is both physical and emotional can then give way to a feeling of empowerment. But before the impulses become visible and we can accompany clients in finishing their incomplete action patterns, they must take possession of their body.

From an evolutionary perspective there are good reasons to suppress impulses to flee or fight in hopeless danger situations so that there are better chances of survival. Our instinct "knows" about this potential dangerous situation and ensures through immobility that we do not have to give in to it. When people have had threatening experiences in their younger years, they become accustomed to suppressing their impulses. Over time, this leads to them no longer feeling these impulses, and experiencing themselves as self-efficient. If we offer an "impulse-friendly" therapy setting, impulses can once again come to light. Then they may be more easily perceived as action or movement impulses, implemented, and finished.

The first step of noticing impulses can consist of clients beginning to make corrections instead of getting stuck in a posture/movement or carrying it out mechanically if they are reluctant or feel uncomfortable. They perceive themselves and their actions as effective and expedient. Here is an example from practice to explain this.

CASE EXAMPLE: YOGA IN A GROUP

I practiced yoga with a group of five women. Each had blankets and pillows available to them, which they could use as they liked. I let them know that they were free to get these aids at any time. I suggested that they check to see whether it would be more comfortable for them to place a pillow under their feet if they felt that the chair was too high. Although two of the women were very short and visibly uncomfortable, they responded with: "No, no, this is alright."

Two weeks later, I noticed how one of the women put a pillow under her feet. Two more followed her example. They noticed their uncomfortable posture and gave in to the impulse of doing something about it. This gave them a sense of self-efficacy.

With increasing interoceptive awareness, the perception becomes more differentiated. The richer the clients' experiences are with the different variations of yoga *asanas*, the more likely it is that they can make a choice and follow an impulse that tells them: "This is good for me, this helps me; I don't like this, I can refrain from this; or I can do something about this." If clients are increasingly capable of noticing their impulses and translating them into action, they gradually touch on their defensive strategies.

Impulses require time. In yoga practice this means that we invite clients to stay in a pose that is pleasant to them until an inner impulse says that they should change this posture. The impetus is not based on a thought, but arises from the feeling that it is good now and something else is even better, or that it is enough now and something new should occur.

At this point, I would like to again quote Norbert Klinkenberg, who relates the idea of the impulse to our everyday life:

> In everyday life, activities and experiences usually don't have an opportunity to fully be effective within us since we are already involved in the next activity. We end an action by already having started the next one, and virtually stumble into the new one without really being ready for it. At the same time, the human structure demands that the things we do are allowed to have effects and that we are also ready for what we want to do. (2007, p.44)

CASE EXAMPLE: LYNETTE

In one session, Lynette sits with her eyes closed in Staff Pose. This allows her to be relaxed as she sits. She then abruptly opens her eyes and draws her legs closer to her.

DH: Hmmm...did you already have enough of Staff Pose?

Lynette: No, but I thought that I should turn back to you again. After all, I can't sit like this forever...

DH: You could try the following. Stay in Staff Pose until an inner impulse tells you that you would like to get into a different posture. This may take a few breaths or maybe a minute... You will sense when the time for a change has come.

DH: If you like, you can continue with the movement... or pause for a moment...and direct your focus to your hands...

Sandra pauses, rubs her hands over her thighs, and sighs.

Sandra: Better...

She continues to stroke her hands over her thighs. I confirm her perception and mirror her movements.

DH: Hmmm... Better...

Sandra: Yes, the warmth of my hands on my thighs feels good to me...

DH: Perhaps your warm hands would also be helpful to your shoulders? If you like, grasp your opposite shoulder or tense muscles with one hand...or gently massage it...

Sandra puts her left hand on the place between her shoulder and neck, the trapezius muscle. I can clearly see that her shoulder lowers slightly after a while. She massages the muscle with her fingers.

Sandra: Very hard...but this feels good...

We stay with this act of self-care for a while. Then Sandra massages her other shoulder and the lowering of the shoulder is also unmistakable. Her facial expression becomes a bit softer.

I suggest a side bend as the next *asana*. The idea is that the shoulder and arm musculature is activated in this position and clients are able to notice a lessening of tension in this area.

DH: Perhaps you would like to try another *asana* that activates your shoulder muscles.

Sandra nods, and I show her the side bend with stretched arms.

DH: You can just stretch one arm upward...like this...and let the other hang down loosely... Or you can bring up both arms...as you bend to the side. How far you bend is up to you.

Sandra decides on both arms and bends to the left.

DH: Perhaps you get an especially clear sense of the muscles in your right shoulder...perhaps also the weight of your arms...or something entirely different... You decide how long you still want to stay in the *asana*—perhaps for another two to three breaths... You can end the *asana* at any time.

Sandra lowers her arms and centers herself.

DH: If you like, you can take a moment and sense how the tension is leaving your muscles.

Sandra: My shoulders now feel much heavier...and so do my arms...and warmer... This is pleasant when the tension decreases. I feel pleasantly tired...

Her breath becomes deeper and her shoulders drop.

The relaxing of muscles has a positive effect on emotional states since, from the bottom up, the body sends signals to the brain that there is no danger.

EXPOSURE AND HABITUATION IN BODY-ORIENTED THERAPY

According to the model of the fear network, all of the triggers—no matter whether they are internal such as emotions, thoughts, physical sensations, and bodily reactions, or external such as sounds, words, people, places, or objects—can set off a stimuli–reaction system. As in a domino effect, the entire fear network is activated, although this is a learned reaction that can be unlearned once again. Edna Foa and colleagues (2000, 2007) use this insight in Prolonged Exposure Therapy (PE). Instead of supporting the avoidance of stimuli, they strive for habituation of the memory stimuli through repeated exposure.

But if the stimuli cannot be tolerated, this makes habituation through the memory of what has happened more difficult. In addition, not everything is so easy to grasp and expose, for example, what is missing or deficiencies. And this is precisely what is involved in cases of neglect, which tend to be the rule instead of the exception in early complex relationship trauma.

What remains is the body, which always has a story to tell. We only need to "listen" to it.

So how can we support clients in giving up their avoidance on the somatic level, and how can habituation to physical sensations and emotions also be achieved when no concrete memories exist?

Although the therapeutic work with TSY doesn't push the trauma exposure into the foreground, we must assume that it can also be awakened through body-oriented work on trauma memories. After an initial stabilization phase in which an effort is made to avoid high states of arousal, clients are supported in noticing their somatic triggers, so the body and its sensations can no longer be ignored. As we know, avoidance thwarts a new corrective learning experience. This is why therapists equip clients with tools to allow them to reduce their reactivity in relation to the trauma triggers through actions and possibilities for relaxation. In TSY, clients are supported in directing awareness to their somatic experience of a trigger with the help of mindfulness, so that habituation can slowly arise. A female client confirms this:

> The first time that you suggested to me that I should bend forward in an *asana*, I was very nervous. It frightened me and I was immensely angry at you for doing that to me. Everything within me resisted. I felt my heart hammering in my entire body and thought for a moment that I couldn't stand it anymore. What helped was that I had my eyes open and you had said time and again that we could keep our eyes open. And your voice, which guided me. It wasn't quite as bad next time. Although my heart was still beating as wildly as always, this was not quite as intense as the first time. That gave me a lot of confidence.

New learning only functions when we work in the "window of tolerance," the area in which sympathetic activation is tolerable for clients, and a parasympathetic shut-down does not occur. This requires activation of the sympathetic nervous system, whereby we once again find ourselves in the area that Marsha Linehan defined in her classification of the stress level as being "between 30 and 70 percent." However, the activation may only go so far that the affected person can tolerate the stress.

So let's come back to the creation of a fear network once again. What occurs on the somatic level in the meantime?

From all of the sensory information, our body constantly chooses where we must direct our attention and what can stay ignored. Emotional reactions to past sensory stimuli influence our relationship to the current similar stimuli through so-called priming. This means that a former stimulus is activated due to previous experiences of usually unconscious implicit memory contents. A word, image, smell, gesture, movement, or even immobility can be such a primed stimulus. This activates memory contents from the bottom up, which are, in turn, processed top down and influence the frame of mind, thoughts, and subsequent behavior, among other things.

While priming protects healthy people from having to constantly re-evaluate an abundance of impressions, this has a dysfunctional effect on trauma clients. During the traumatic event they absorb the stimuli that later remind them of these horrible things. All of the information that could help them to differentiate between a current situation and the one at the time has been filtered out (see Ogden *et al.* 2006, p.57ff.). The therapeutic goal is therefore to implant information that gives clients a feeling for the present, the here and now, in a state of high arousal. They should be able to recognize that the "past" feelings and situations have been experienced, but that they are currently in a completely different context. This perception—which is experienced less cognitively than somatically—helps clients to better tolerate feelings and memories.

To start with I wasn't always successful in translating these perceptions in the therapy and the here and now with my voice, or anchoring it through orientation in space in the hope that the clients could create a relationship with the present. I therefore rely on interoceptive resources today. I illustrate this again here by using an example from my practice in a later session with Sandra. One trigger catapulted her into her traumatic past, and the familiar panic spread within her that took her breath away.

CASE EXAMPLE: SANDRA

DH: If you feel your feet on the floor at this moment... perhaps even look down at them...move your toes...while you slide your feet across the floor... [I comment what I see here] then you are in the now as you simultaneously notice these feelings from your past.

The somatic resources of "contact with the feet on the floor" had by now become a reliable anchor that Sandra also frequently used in her everyday life, and represented an adequate counterbalance to the pull of the trauma.

Sandra moves her feet across the floor and then looks at me in complete surprise.

Sandra: This may sound banal, and I've already thought and knew this before, but now I've felt it for the first time. I'm here and sense feelings from the past—not what is happening right now. This feels completely different!

DH: I'm certain that you have frequently thought this already and also absolutely comprehended it cognitively, but it hadn't arrived in your body up to now. Now it has slid down from your head to your belly.

Sandra: Exactly. How often have I thought: "Don't make such a fuss. After all, you know that this is no longer relevant and that you're an adult now" and so forth. But these thoughts oppressed me even more. Seeing and feeling my feet is definitely something that belongs in the present.

For the first time, she succeeds in expanding her filter during an arousal and absorbing information to show her that she is in a completely different situation now.

Any stimulus that is picked up and processed through sensory impressions leads to physical and emotional reactions due to priming. In order for trauma clients to even perceive the interoceptive physical signals as such, they require practice in mindful observation on a low level of arousal. This is the only way that the primary goal—implementation of new primings—can be achieved.

In many cases, cognitive knowledge is not enough to stop the arousal. The priming is anchored in the subcortical brain structures, and insight alone can't change them. But if a perception leads to a change in physical and emotional sensing, this also creates new primings that are controlled from the top down.

I like to explain the dissolution of a trigger to my clients with a vivid example: We can make good progress on a well-developed six-lane freeway. By contrast, new priming is comparable with a path that has been cut through the jungle with a machete. If it is rarely used, nature quickly reconquers it. Then we can only make slow and tedious progress. It only becomes a beaten track when used more frequently, then a hiking trail, and a country road, through frequent use. At the same time, the "renaturation" of the freeway starts because it is used less and less frequently. It takes some time for the new path to become a habit.

If we translate this into practicing yoga together, we leave the old pathways and instead establish new priming in the body. Through this mindful sensing and perceiving, the information that is normally overlooked can reach the conscious mind. A movement activates an arousal. At the same time, clients feel that their feet—unimpressed by the state of alarm—give them support. A posture reminds them of the emotional stupor, but they notice that they can move at the same moment.

A RELATIONSHIP OF EQUALS

A relationship of equals is the sharing of experiences that are expressed in a relaxed and emotionally secure setting through a harmony of gestures, facial expressions, movements, pitch, etc. In a relationship trauma, precisely the opposite happens. This is not about the sharing of an experience; it involves the satisfaction of needs of one individual at the cost of the other, whether this is through abuse—where one person takes advantage of the other—or through neglect—where the needs of one person cannot be brought into harmony with those of the other.

A relationship trauma can also be seen as a non-reflected mirroring. In keeping with our age, we express a refusal in either a verbal or non-verbal way.

The more we are attuned to another person, the more distinctly we mirror each other. In turn, this leads to more connectedness. This process creates a rhythm or dance that happens virtually on its own and that we register unconsciously. This rhythm is disturbed in people who suffer from complex trauma. The unconscious mirroring and leading no longer takes place. They can no longer attune their movements and facial expressions to other people.

When I began to work with trauma clients, I was irritated when they sat across from me as stiff as statues, or collapsed within themselves, showing little feeling or facial expressions. There was the client and me, both of us completely disconnected from each other. Practically no smile and no expression of anger or concern, not even the slightest sign of accord or even the disparities that normally wander back and forth. For my part, I started mirroring the displayed or, more precisely, the not displayed, body movements and facial expressions. Then I began to observe my own feelings and sensations. This allowed me to get an insight into the state of the affected person in terms of what it means to be in a body that is frozen in the moment of trauma. I became aware of how tense I was, how superficial my breath was, and how helpless and stressed I felt because my offers and desires for a relationship remained unfulfilled.

Differentiating this pacing (mirroring) from my own tension is an important step for the differentiation of a person's own emotions and sensations. One is a deliberately created state, while we can "slide" into the other. Being able to consciously relax, take a deep breath, and reflect mindfully on the present moment is the best thing that we can do for ourselves and for our clients. By observing what this feeling of unrelatedness does to us, we can scale back our own needs so that we do not fall into the trap of non-verbally subjecting our clients to pressure with our desire for a relationship. This is an important aspect in creating a relationship with traumatized clients. If we do not respect this, we may conjure up the danger of repeating the same drama on a different stage. When I expanded my therapy approach by offering body-oriented exercises, a path opened up for me to offer resonance and commonality without a relationship or the desire for a relationship. As a result, there was no demand on the clients.

I won't go into more detail here about the phenomenon of mirror neurons (cf. Bauer 2006; Damasio 2006; Rizzolatti and Craighero 2004). Just this: Mirror neurons have the effect that, through the observation of our counterpart, the same motor and emotional reactions are triggered within us. We can make use of this when we practice together. Clients who are hardly able to perceive their body or parts of it get the chance to orient themselves on us, and simultaneously experience something about themselves by observing the same movement and posture.

If we want to make it possible for clients to engage in sharing experiences and mirroring, we must strive for a relationship on an equal basis. If we enter into a space together with the clients in which we do the same movements or breathing techniques, and mirror our personal, interoceptive perceptions, we find ourselves in our very own experiential space of self-perception in our human body—together and simultaneously, individually, on our own. These experiences could not differ more from a traumatic experience. Relationships that may otherwise remind someone of previous "abuse" can be experienced in this way without demands. And because clients are also not left alone, no experience of "neglect" can arise. They experience harmony and pacing. On the other hand, even well intended establishing of contact and asking questions may trigger major stress in clients, which is an experience that I have had. In this case, clients feel that they are once again in a situation of powerlessness, helplessly at someone's mercy. Either explicitly or implicitly, they are reminded of their trauma experience. To better understand this, here is a brief excerpt from a session with Frances.

CASE EXAMPLE: FRANCES

Since Frances noticed that she repeatedly felt depressed and weak, we decided on some activating standing *asana*s in this session. After we set up the Warrior Poses together and explored them, I suggested that she loosen her shoulders... and circle them a bit...observe the circle movements...also by looking at her shoulders... Or clasp each of the shoulders with a hand and circle the elbows... Frances tries both variations.

Frances: When I see my shoulders circling, it becomes easier to feel the movement. When I have my eyes closed, I sense less. What surprises me is that I feel my shoulders and muscles better when I observe how your shoulders move.

DH: This is interesting... Then it is sometimes good to practice with open eyes and observe how I move my shoulders.

in which we repeatedly use words such as "can," "power," "decide," "choose," etc. If clients feel that they are mastering something real as they do this, this is also reflected in their observation and feelings. A female client expressed it like this: "You can't tell me often enough that I can make a choice. At the beginning of the therapy, I felt that this was frightening. It no longer bothers me, but I still tend to forget it."

I am convinced that our words can only have an effect when our clients experience these words as honest, and that we don't project any false facts through them. So when we accompany the process of interoceptive perception and repeatedly focus on the idea that clients can stop at any time, direct their attention to something else, change a posture, and are allowed to refuse our suggestions, this will become their world of experience and felt reality. Yet a word of warning is appropriate here. If we praise clients, some will just presumably use the options to which they are accustomed—doing what others expect of them. Not choosing is just as appropriate as choosing!

In body-oriented work I have quite frequently observed that beliefs change without us explicitly speaking about them.

CASE EXAMPLE: FRANCES

Frances was completely distraught as she came to the session. The traumatic memories that had appeared during the previous night had caused her to tremble and turn as white as a sheet. In accordance with her wishes, we begin with yoga in Mountain Pose. However, the state of her arousal reaches the highest level on a scale of 0–10, and this can no longer be tamed just through sitting. I remind her of the effect that the Sun Breath has. We practice together for quite some time, and she gradually starts to calm down.

As she does this, she keeps her eyes closed while I occasionally comment on the movements and the breath with "inhale and exhale," as well as encourage her with "exactly" or "great" so that I don't lose contact with her.

Frances: I'm now at level 3 in terms of relaxation. But my fear has simultaneously increased to level 7.

DH: Perhaps there's a difference between whether your eyes are open or closed...

My hypothesis was that the closed eyes increase her fear, which Frances confirms.

Frances: The fear comes down to level 4 when I open my eyes. This is a bit less relaxed and no longer quite as pleasant.

DH: This means that you can choose whether you want to tolerate the fear and enjoy more relaxation as a result, or whether you are willing to somewhat let go of this beautiful sense of relaxation and feel less fear.

At this point, it's important to me to use words such as "choose" and "decide." I want to make Frances aware that she is not at the mercy of her affects and that she can very well influence something.

Frances tries it briefly by opening her eyes and closing them. Then she stays in Mountain Pose with opened eyes.

Frances: Now I prefer to have less fear.

Some sessions later, she uses her newly acquired ability and opens her eyes on her own as the flood of memories becomes too much for her. She reports to me how good it feels to be able to influence something and that she now no longer assumes that she is helplessly and powerlessly at the mercy of every situation.

The bottom-up changes of beliefs often occur almost unnoticed. I sometimes hear a client talk about circumstances in which they act completely differently from some weeks ago, and they often don't even notice this. Their successes and achievements only become clear when we address them.

REDUCING STATES OF TENSION IN THE BODY

Gentle and calming *asanas* are not helpful in every case. An example from my practice shows that, in some cases, this may even be counterproductive at the start of the therapy.

CASE EXAMPLE: HELEN

Helen had been abused for years when she was young, and tended to engage in self-injury in order to relieve her tension. After a hospital stay, she made an appointment with me so she could come to terms with her traumatic childhood experiences.

In the first hour, she sits trembling and tense in front of me. Her hands are interwoven with each other and her legs tightly crossed. Her entire body is in a state of high tension. She avoids any type of eye contact. After a phase of getting to know each other and psychoeducation—in which I explain my body-oriented approach to her—I suggest that we search for something that helps her to reduce her tension. It was important to me that we find something before working with the traumatic contents. My worry was that she could begin hurting herself more again if I start exposure therapy too soon.

I introduce a scale of 0–10 for her tension right at the start so that we can both learn what leads to a reduction of tension and what causes increased activation. Helen can hardly tolerate even just this conversation about the approach of the trauma therapy and the prospect of resurrecting the past once again. But we haven't even started in terms of working on the content yet.

I suggest to her that she sits on the yoga chair and feels her feet, moves them, etc., in order to set up Mountain Pose in small steps. When we reach the shoulders and I ask her to feel what changes, she senses when moving her shoulders a bit that her tension increases.

Helen: Moving my shoulders makes me vulnerable. That doesn't work at all.

She is extremely tense in the upper area of her body and bends forward again.

I try a Cat–Cow movement, which can give her a sense of empowerment to make her own choice. But this also doesn't bring any relief—quite the opposite, in fact.

Helen gladly accepts my suggestion to stand up and try a few powerful *asanas*. We start with Warrior Pose I and II and then continue with Powerful Pose, Downward Dog, and Three-Legged Dog Pose. To get some reassurance, I ask her several times during the practice how she evaluates her tension. It initially falls from 7 to 5 and even goes down to 2 in the further course of the practice.

Since Helen is very athletic and primarily attempts to reduce her tension through fast running and cycling, the exercises are not difficult for her. However, I sometimes have difficulty keeping up with her. This has the positive effect that I am repeatedly the one who has to give up. This allows me to encourage her in selecting an appropriate time span. This situation sometimes makes us laugh and creates moments of relaxation. At the same time, Helen experiences through my role model that I practice without any ambitions, take care of myself, and don't ask too much of myself—which are implicit messages, as described by Gerbarg (2008).

In the following session, she once again sits trembling and tense in front of me—"on a 6–7," according to her estimate—and we immediately start with the strengthening *asanas*. Once she has reached a 3, we can enter into a conversation and begin speaking about her childhood in general. Since her tension continuously increases during the conversation, we repeatedly switch back and forth between the *asanas* and talking. In this way, a rhythm of tension— through remembering her childhood (not the traumas)—and relaxation develops while practicing the *asanas*.

We are able to begin the third session with somewhat less tension (3–4); this time, Helen is even quite relaxed as she sits across from me. Knowing that her tension can be controlled and regulated at any time makes us both feel more secure. In the course of the following sessions, we draw on both the dynamic *asanas* and the Bellows Breath. This makes it possible for Helen to get her tension under control.

The case examples in this chapter clearly show that therapists are not the experts. We can't know which *asana* or breathing exercise is the right "medicine." Only the clients themselves can find out how to calm their states of tension, activations, and arousals. If we are ready to encounter them on an equal basis and to allow ourselves to be guided by the experiences of our clients, this creates a field in which they can try things out, reject them, and make a fresh attempt—until the result is satisfactory. This makes it possible to have an experience that is diametrically opposed to the traumatization.

CONCLUDING
THOUGHTS

Out beyond ideas of wrongdoing and rightdoing there is a field. I'll meet you there.

When the soul lies down in that grass the world is too full to talk about.

Ideas, language, even the phrase "each other" doesn't make any sense. (Rumi 1995)

I would now like to once again return to the question, "Can yoga be a substitute for trauma therapy?"

If I look at my daily practice, the answer is clearly "no." I am convinced that people need both therapy and yoga, to help them at a cognitive and emotional level, as well as physically. This is only possible with a conversation about the trauma and its consequences. Listening, empathy, compassion, and understanding are just as important as cognitive understanding and being able to make links.

If we understand a successful trauma therapy as simply the reduction of PTSD symptoms, this could—as convincingly proven by various studies—be enough for those affected to attend a TSY group. But particularly in clients who have suffered from complex trauma, we primarily see disorders in the area of attachment relationships and the "destruction" of important aspects in their lives due to these experiences. So we can't avoid speaking with our clients about their losses, the betrayal that they were perhaps subjected to, their incomprehension, and their hopelessness. By taking their pain, fears, suffering, anger, helplessness, and grief seriously, and acknowledging these as compassionate and empathetic counterparts, we allow all of these emotions to exist. If we help them to understand why they have become as they are, they may gradually comprehend that it isn't their fault and that they don't need to be ashamed of their feelings. This is how we can accompany our clients so that they are able to see the past as being over but able to look at the future as something that can be shaped as it lies ahead of them and offers them opportunities.

Before clients can deal with the feelings of anger, blame, or grief, a trauma exposure must occur in most cases. This helps to counteract the avoidance that is standing in the way of working through the trauma. It addresses habituation and helps clients have new learning experiences and insights. This makes it an important element of a successful trauma therapy.

However, in order to even bear a trauma exposure and to be able to talk about experiences, feelings, and effects, we need tools to help clients get control of their affects and physical reactions. Within this context, conversations are less useful than a body-oriented way of working. Through a careful approach, clients become capable of tolerating trauma-related triggers, which are expressed as physical symptoms. This allows them to feel an arousal and to successfully stop it. The same also applies to a shut-down. As a result, clients achieve control over their emotions and sensations.

This brings us to the three steps of trauma therapy: stabilization, trauma exposure, and integration. My intention with this book is to put a body-related touch into the stabilization phase. This is based less on developing a relationship with the other person; instead, the intention is for an individual to create a relationship with themselves and with their own body. This can work with physical exercises, which are offered in a multitude of variations by yoga. Once stabilization has been achieved, there is no longer anything standing in the way of trauma exposure and integration.

In one of his lectures, Bessel van der Kolk expressed this as follows: In the trauma work with yoga, we focus on relationship of the clients with their body and not—as in the therapy—their relationship with us (2014 lecture, during a five-day advanced training in TSY).

If we open up Rumi's field in which there is no idea of right or wrong and meet our clients there, the following becomes possible. Through interoceptive perception and self-exploration, clients can begin to create a relationship with their own self, take possession of their body, and gradually notice what they like and what allows them to feel good, as well as what they don't want and what they can change or reject as a result. In the relationship with their self they will find the stability that allows them to face their traumatic past.

APPENDIX

QUESTIONNAIRE FOLLOWING A YOGA COURSE

I would be pleased if you could take a moment to answer the questions below. Your feedback will let me know what was good for you and/or helped you, and what I can do better.

Thank you very much!

Please think back to the time before the yoga course, and briefly describe the long-term effects that your traumatic experiences had on you and your life. This may be in relation to emotions, physical sensations, thoughts about yourself and the world, the future, your relationship with your body, your relationship with the community, or connections with other people.

_____

_____

_____

_____

Have these effects that were caused by the traumatic experiences improved, have they remained the same, or have they worsened?

_____

_____

Which (new) experiences did you have in the yoga classes? These can be either positive or negative.

_____

_____

Have you noticed any type of changes (with regard to thoughts, emotions, physical sensations, your relationship with your body, and your relationship with people around you) during your participation in the yoga? If yes, which?

_____

_____

_____

_____

Have you had particularly *positive* experiences such as an especially good moment or an aspect during the yoga course or due to your participation in the yoga course?

_____

_____

Have you had particularly *negative* experiences such as an especially difficult moment or an aspect during the yoga course or due to your participation in the yoga course?

_____

_____

What else would you like to tell me?

_____

_____

_____

QUESTIONNAIRE ON THE EFFECT OF THE YOGA PRACTICE

Week: _____   Date: _____

In order to document your success, it is a good idea to briefly pause once a week to determine what has changed for you due to your yoga practice.

Which (new) experiences (positive or negative) have you had during the past week in your yoga practice?

_____

_____

Emotions:

_____

_____

Physical sensations:

_____

_____

Thoughts about yourself and the world:

_____

_____

Thoughts about the future:

_____

_____

Your relationship with your body:

_____

_____

Your relationship with other people:

_____

_____

Have you noticed any type of changes while practicing yoga? If *yes,* which?

_____

_____

Did you have especially *positive* experiences, an especially good moment or aspect during the past week?

_____

_____

Did you have especially *negative* experiences, an especially difficult moment or aspect during the past week?

_____

_____

What else did you notice?

_____

_____

HANDOUT—MAKING CONTACT WITH YOUR BODY

We start in seated Mountain Pose.

Take a moment to arrange yourself on your chair so that you are sitting comfortably. For Mountain Pose, you can place your feet at hip width apart or a little wider or narrower—whatever feels good for you.

Put your feet very consciously on the floor; perhaps also take a brief look at the position of your feet. When you are ready, make contact with the floor in your own way by either feeling the weight of your feet on the floor, or by lifting your feet and moving them across the floor, or doing something your own way.

Stay with the feeling of contact with the floor for one to three breaths.

Now bring your attention to the middle of your body, in the area of your navel and the lower part of your back. You can deepen the contact with the middle of your body by placing one hand on your belly, for example. You can strengthen your perception of your back by leaning on the backrest of your chair.

Stay in the feeling of contact in the middle of your body for one to three breaths.

You could also straighten your body and let your spinal column "grow" in the direction of the ceiling, to generate a feeling of length in your body.

Take the time of one to three breaths for this sensation.

If you have had your eyes closed up to now, gently open them and get comfortable on your chair.

YOGA NOTES

When you practice yoga by yourself, it can be helpful to write down what you have noticed on a regular basis so that you can discuss these findings in the therapy.

1. Is there an area of your body or a sensation that you noticed while you practiced? If yes, what was it and how did you notice it?

_____

_____

_____

_____

_____

_____

2. Did you notice something in relation to your breath while you practiced?

_____

_____

_____

_____

_____

3. While you practiced, did you allow yourself to try something out, make changes, or make use of choice?

_____

_____

_____

_____

References

Adkins, C.C., Robinson, O.B., and Stewart, B.L. (2011) *Chair Yoga for You: A Practical Guide.* CreateSpace Independent Publishing Platform. Library of Congress Control Number 2010916650.

APA (American Psychiatric Association) (2000) *Diagnostic and Statistical Manual of Mental Disorders, 4th edn, Text Revision (DSM-IV).* Washington, DC: APA.

APA (2013) *Diagnostic and Statistical Manual of Mental Disorders, 5th edn (DSM-5).* Arlington, VA: APA. Available at www.dsm5.org/psychiatrists/practice/dsm, accessed on 9 January 2017.

Arch, J.J. and Craske, M.G. (2006) 'Mechanism of mindfulness: Emotion regulation following a focused breathing induction.' *Behaviour Research and Therapy 44,* 1849–58.

Baer, R.A. (2003) 'Mindfulness training as a clinical intervention: A conceptual and empirical review.' *Clinical Psychology: Science and Practice 10,* 125–43.

Bauer, J. (2006) *Warum ich Fühle, Was du Fühlst. Intuitive Kommunikation und das Geheimnis der Spiegelneuronen [Why I Feel What You Feel: Intuitive Communication and the Secret of Mirror Neurons].* Hamburg: Hoffmann & Campe.

Begley, S. (2010) *Neue Gedanken—Neues Gehirn: Die Wissenschaft der neuroplastizität Beweist, Wie unser Bewusstsein das Gehirn verändert.* Munich: Goldmann.

Behanan, Kovoor T. Yog (1937) *A Scientific Evaluation.* New York: Macmillan.

Bernardi, L., Porta, C., Gabutti, A., Spicuzza, L., and Sleigt, P. (2001) 'Modulatory effects of respiration.' *Autonomic Neuroscience 90*(1–2), 47–56.

Berrol, C. F. (1992) 'The neurophysiologic basis of the mind-body connection in dance/movement therapy.' *American Journal of Dance Therapy 14*(2), 19–29.

Bhargava, R., Gogate, M.G., and Mascarenhas, J.F. (1988) 'Autonomic responses to breath holding and its variations following pranayama.' *Indian Journal of Physiology and Pharmacology 32,* 257–64.

Bishop, S.R., Lau, M., Shapiro, S., Carlson, L. *et al.* (2004) 'Mindfulness: A proposed operational definition.' *Clinical Psychology: Science and Practice 11,* 230–41.

Brewin, C.R., Dagleish, T., and Joseph, S. (1996) 'A dual representation theory of post-traumatic stress disorder.' *Psychological Review 103,* 670–86.

Broad, W.J. (2012) *The Science of Yoga. Was es Verspricht—und Was es Kann.* Freiburg: Herder.

Brown, K.W. and Ryan, R.M. (2003) 'The benefits of being present: Mindfulness and its role in psychological well-being.' *Journal of Personality and Social Psychology 84,* 822–48.

Brown, K.W., Ryan, R.M., and Creswell, J.D. (2007) 'Mindfulness: Theoretical foundations and evidence for its salutary effects.' *Psychological Inquiry 18, 4, 211–237.*

Brown, R.P. and Gerbarg, P.L. (2009) 'Yoga breathing, meditation, and longevity.' *Longevity, Regeneration, and Optimal Health: Annals of New York Academy of Science 1172,* 54–62.

Cahn, B.R. and Polich, J. (2006) 'Meditation states and traits: EEG, ERP, and neuroimaging studies.' *Psychological Bulletin 132,* 180–211.

Cappo, B.M. and Holmes, D.S. (1984) 'The utility of prolonged respiration exhalation for reducing physiological and psychological arousal in non-threatening and threatening situations.' *Journal of Psychosomatic Research 28,* 265–73.

Carter, J.J. and Byrne, G.G. (2004) 'A two year study of the use of yoga in a series of pilot studies as an adjunct to ordinary psychiatric treatment in a group of Vietnam War veterans suffering from posttraumatic stress disorder.' Available at www. therapywithyoga.com/Vivekananda.pdf.

Carter, J.J. and Byrne, G.G. (2006) 'PTSD Australian Vietnam veterans: Yoga adjunct treatment two RCTs: MCYI and SKY.' Proceedings of the World Conference 'Expanding Paradigms: Science, Consciousness and Spirituality Proceedings', February. New Delhi, India: All India Institute of Medical Sciences.

Catani, C., Kohiladevy, M., Ruf, M., Schauer, E., Elbert, T., and Neuner F. (2009) 'Treating children traumatized by war and tsunami: A comparison between exposure therapy and meditation-relaxation in North-East Sri Lanka.' *BMC Psychiatry 9,* 22.

Coulter, D.H. (2009) *Anatomie des Hatha Yoga. Ein Handbuch für Schüler, Lehrer und Praktizierende.* Yoga Verlag GmbH.

Crisan, H.G. (1984) Pranayama in Anxiety Neurosis—A Pilot Study. MD dissertation submitted to the University of Heidelberg, Germany.

D'Andrea, W., Ford, J., Stolbach, B., Spinazzola, J., and van der Kolk, B.A. (2012) 'Understanding interpersonal trauma in children: Why we need a developmentally appropriate trauma diagnosis.' *American Journal of Orthopsychiatry 82*(2), 187–200.

Damasio, A. (2006) *Ich fühle, also bin ich: Die Entschlüsselung des Bewusstseins.* München: List Verlag.

Daubenheimer, J.J. (2005) 'The relationship of yoga, body awareness, and body responsiveness to self-objectification and disordered eating.' *Psychology of Women Quarterly 29,* 207–19.

Delgado, L.C., Guerra, P., Perakakis, P., Vera, M., del Paso, G.R., and Vila, J. (2010) 'Treating chronic worry: Psychological and physiological effects of a training programme based on mindfulness.' *Behavior Research and Therapy 48,* 873–82.

Descilo, T., Vedamurtachar, A., Gerbarg, P.L., Nagaraja, D. *et al.* (2010) 'Effects of a yoga breath intervention alone and in combination with an exposure therapy for posttraumatic stress disorder and depression in survivors of the 2004 South-East Asia tsunami.' *Acta Psychiatrica Scandinavica 121,* 289–300.

Dispenza J. (2009) *Evolve Your Brain: The Science of Changing Your Mind.* Deerfield Beach, FL: Health Communications.

Ehlers, A. (1999) *Posttraumatische Belastungsstörung.* Göttingen: Hogrefe.

Ehlers, A. and Clark D. (2000) 'A cognitive model of posttraumatic stress disorder.' *Behaviour Research and Therapy 38*(4), 19–45.

Ekman, P., Davidson, R.J., Ricard, M., and Wallace, B.A. (2005) 'Buddhist and psychological perspectives on emotions and well-being.' *Current Directions in Psychological Science 14,* 59–63.

Emerson, D. (2012) 'Interview: Yoga teachers as part of the clinical team.' *Yoga Therapy Today,* 24–5.

Emerson, D. and Hopper, E. (2011) *Overcoming Trauma Through Yoga: Reclaiming Your Body.* Berkeley, CA: North Atlantic Books.

Emerson, D., Sharma, R., Chaudhry, S., and Turner J. (2009) 'Yoga therapy in practice: Trauma-sensitive yoga: Principles, practice, and research.' *International Journal of Yoga Therapy 19*, 123–8.

Engel, K. (1999) *Meditation: Geschichte, Systematik, Forschung, Theorie.* Peter Lang: Frankfurt am Main.

Faulds, R. (2005) *Kripalu Yoga. A Guide to Practice On and Off the Mat.* New York: Bantam Dell.

Felitti, V.J. and Anda, R.F. (1997) *The Adverse Childhood Experience (ACE) Study.* Atlanta, GA: Centers for Disease Control and Prevention. Available at www.cdc.gov/ace/index.htm, accessed on 6 January 2017.

Figley, C.R. (2002) *Brief Treatments for the Traumatized. A Project of the Green Cross Foundation.* Westport, CT: Greenwood Press.

Fisher, A., Murray, E., and Bundy, A. (1991) *Sensory Integration Theory and Practice.* Philadelphia, PA: F.A. Davis & Company.

Foa, E.B., Hembree, E.A., and Rothbaum, B.O. (2007) 'Prolonged Exposure Therapy for PTSD: Emotional Processing Therapy of Traumatic Experiences. Therapist Guide.' In P.E. Nathan and J.M. Gorman (eds) *A Guide to Treatments that Work.* New York: Oxford University Press.

Foa, E.B., Keane, T., and Friedman, M.J. (eds) (2000) *Treatment Guidelines for Posttraumatic Stress Disorder.* New York: Guilford Press.

Fogel, A. (2009) *Selbstwahrnehmung und Embodiment in der Körperpsychotherapie: Vom Körpergefühl zur Kognition.* Stuttgart: Schattauer.

Ford, J.D., Grasso, D., Greene, C., Levine, J., Spinazzola, J., and van der Kolk, B. (2013) 'Clinical significance of a proposed developmental trauma disorder diagnosis: Results of an international survey of clinicians.' *Journal of Clinical Psychiatry 74*(8), 841–9.

Franzblau, S.H., Smith, M., Echevarria, S., and van Cantfort, T.E. (2006) 'Take a breath, break the silence: The effects of yogic breathing and testimony about battering on feelings of self-efficacy in battered women.' *International Journal of Yoga Therapy 16*(1), 49–57.

Fuchs, C. (2007) *Die Geschichte des Yoga: Der Weg des Yoga.* Petersberg: Verlag Via Nova.

Fuchs, T. (2008) *Das Gehirn—Ein Beziehungsorgan: Eine phänomenologische-ökologische Konzeption.* Stuttgart: Kohlhammer.

Gerbarg, P.L. (2008) 'Yoga and Neuro-Psychoanalysis.' In F. Anderson (ed.) *Bodies in Treatment: The Unspoken Dimension* (pp.127–50). New York: The Analytic Press.

Glover, D. (2006) 'Psychobiology of posttraumatic stress disorder: A decade of progress.' *Annals of the New York Academy of Sciences 1071*, 442–47.

Goldstein, B.E. (2007) *Wahrnehmungspsychologie: Der Grundkurs.* Heidelberg: Spectrum Verlag.

Goleman, D. (2003) *The Meditative Mind. The Varieties of Meditative Experience.* New York: G.P. Putnam's & Sons.

Graubner, B. (2012) *ICD-10-GM 2013 Systematisches Verzeichnis: Internationale Statistische Klassifikation der Krankheiten und Verwandter Gesundheitsprobleme.* Cologne: Deutscher Ärzte-Verlag.

Grawe, K. (2004) *Neuropsychotherapie.* Göttingen: Hogrefe.

Grossmann, K.E. (ed.) (2011) *Bindung und Menschliche Entwicklung: John Bowlby, Mary Ainsworth und die Grundlagen der Bindungstheorie.* Stuttgart: Klett-Cotta.

Hart, W. (1987) *The Art of Living: Vipassana-Meditation as Taught by S. N. Goenka.* San Francisco, CA: Harper & Row.

Hawley, J. (2002) *Bhagavad Gita.* Munich: Goldmann.

Herman, J.L. (2003) *Trauma and Recovery: The Aftermath of Violence—From Domestic Abuse to Political Terror.* New York: Basic Books.

Hölzel, B.K. (2007) Kumulativ-Dissertation zur Erlangung des Doktorgrades der Naturwissenschaften. Dr. rer. nat. Der Fakultät für Naturwissenschaften der Justus-Liebig-Universität Giessen.

Horowitz, M.J. (1974) 'Persönlichkeitsstile und Belastungsfolgen. Integrative Psychodynamisch-kognitive Psychotherapie.' In A. Maercker (1997). *Therapie der Posttraumatischen Belastungsstörungen* (pp.145–79). Berlin: Springer.

Huestegge, L. (2014) 'Top-down-Verarbeitung.' In M.A. Wirtz (ed.) *Dorsch—Lexikon der Psychologie* (16th edn). Bern: Verlag Hans Huber.

Huppertz, M. (2011) *Achtsamkeitsübungen: Experimente mit einem anderen Lebensgefühl.* Paderborn: Junfermann.

Isabella, R.A. and Belsky, J. (1991) 'Interactional synchrony and the origins of infant-mother attachment: A replication study.' *Child Development 62*, 373–84.

Jha, A.P., Krompinger, J., and Baime, M. (2007) 'Mindfulness training modifies subsystems of attention.' *Cognitive, Affective, and Behavioral Neuroscience 7*, 109–19.

Johnston, J. (2011) *The Impact of Yoga on Military Personnel with Posttraumatic Stress Disorder.* Counseling Psychology Dissertations Paper 29. Boston, MA: Northeastern University.

Joseph, R. (1996) *Neuropsychology, Neuropsychiatry, and Behavioral Neurology.* New York: Williams & Wilkins.

Jovanov, E. (2005) 'On Spectral Analysis of Heart Rate Variability During Very Slow Yogic Breathing.' Conference Proceedings: Annual International Conference of the IEEE Engineering in Medicine and Biology Society, 3, 2467–70.

Kabat-Zinn, J. (1990) *Full Catastrophe Living: Using the Wisdom of Your Body and Mind to Face Stress, Pain, and Illness.* New York: Delacorte.

Kabat-Zinn, J. (2007) *Im Alltag Ruhe Finden. Das Umfassende Praktische Meditationsprogramm.* Freiburg: Herder.

Khalsa Dharma Singh and Stauth, C. (2004) *Mediation as Medicine.* New York: Simon & Schuster.

Kisiel, C.L., Fehrenbach, T., Torgersen, E., Stolbach, B. *et al.* (2014) 'Constellations of interpersonal trauma and symptoms in child welfare: Implications for a developmental trauma framework.' *Journal of Family Violence 29*, 1–14.

Kissen, M. and Kissen-Kohn, D. A. (2009) 'Reducing addictions via the self-soothing effects of yoga.' *Bulletin of the Menninger Clinic 73*(1), 34–43.

Klinkenberg, N. (2007) *Achtsamkeit in der Körperverhaltenstherapie.* Stuttgart: Klett-Cotta.

Larsen, S., Yee, W., Gerbarg, P.L., Brown, R.P., Gunkelman, J., and Sherlin, L. (2006) 'Neurophysiological Markers of Sudarshan Kriya Yoga Practitioners: A Pilot Study.' Proceedings of the World Conference 'Expanding Paradigms: Science, Consciousness and Spirituality', 24–25 February. New Delhi, India: All India Institute of Medical Sciences, pp.36–48.

Lazar, S.W., Kerr, C.E., Wasserman, R.H., Gray, J.R. *et al.* (2005) 'Meditation experience is associated with increased cortical thickness.' *Neuroreport 16*, 1893–97.

Lenzen, M. (1997) 'Besprechung von "Descartes Irrtum".' *Spektrum der Wissenschaft*, Mai, p.124.

Lenzinger-Bohleber, M., Roth, G., and Buchheim, A. (2008) *Psychoanalyse, Neurobiologie und Trauma.* Stuttgart: Schattauer.

Levine, P. (1976) *Waking the Tiger: Healing Trauma.* Berkeley, CA: North Atlantic Books.

Levine, P. (2010) *In an Unspoken Voice: How the Body Releases Trauma and Restores Goodness.* Berkeley, CA: North Atlantic Books.

Lilly, M. and Hedlund, J. (2010) 'Yoga therapy in practice. Healing childhood sexual abuse with yoga.' *International Journal of Yoga Therapy 20*, 120–30.

Lueger-Schuster, B. (2008) 'Diagnostik Posttraumatischer Belastungsstörung.' *Psychiatria Danubina 20*(4), 521–31.

Maercker, A. (2009) *Posttraumatische Belastungsstörung*. Berlin: Springer.

Mahasi Sayadaw (1971) *Satipatthana Vipassana: Insight through Mindfulness*. Kandy, Sri Lanka: Buddhist Publication Society.

Meltzoff, A.N. and Moore, M.K. (1983) 'Newborn infants imitate adult facial gestures.' *Child Development 54*, 702–9.

Merleau-Ponty, M. (2004) *The World of Perception*. Abingdon: Routledge.

Merzenich, M.M., Nelson, R.J., Kaas, J.H., Stryker, M.P. *et al.* (1987) 'Variability in hand surface representations in areas 3b and 1 in adult owl and squirrel monkeys.' *Journal of Comparative Neurology 258*(2), 281–96.

Newberg, A.B. and Iversen, J. (2003) 'The neural basis of the complex mental task of meditation: Neurotransmitter and neurochemical considerations.' *Medical Hypotheses 61*, 282–91.

Newlin, C. (2011) *Overview of the Adverse Experiences in Childhood (ACE) Study*. Huntsville, AL: National Children's Advocacy Center.

Niedenthal, P.M., Barsalou, L.W., Fischer, J., Vollmar, P., Heidenreich, T., and Schulte, D. (2009) 'Embodiment on sadness and depression—Gait patterns associated with dysphoric mood.' *Psychosomatic Medicine 71*, 580–87.

Nijenhuis, E.R. (2009) 'Somatoform dissociation and somatoform dissociative disorders.' In P.F. Deli and J. O'Neil (eds) *Dissociation and Dissociative Disorders: DSM-IV and Beyond (pp.245–73)*. New York: Routledge.

Nijenhuis, E.R., van der Hart, O., Kruger, K., and Steele, K. (2004) 'Somatoform dissociation, reported abuse and animal defence-like reactions.' *Australian and New Zealand Journal of Psychiatry 38*(9), 678–86.

Nijenhuis, E.R., Spinhoven, P., van Dyck, R., van der Hart, O., and Vanderlinden, J. (1996) 'The development and psychometric characteristics of the somatoform Dissociation Questionnaire (sDQ-20).' *Journal of Nervous and Mental Disorder 184*(11), 688–94.

Ogden, P. and Minton, K. (2000) 'Sensorimotor psychotherapy: One method for processing traumatic memory.' *Traumatology 6*(3), 149–73.

Ogden, P., Minton, K., and Pain, C. (2006) *Trauma und Körper. Ein Sensumotorisch Orientierter Psychotherapeutischer Ansatz*. Paderborn: Junfermann.

Patanjali (2010) *Die Wurzeln des Yoga: Die Klassischen Lehrsprüche des Pantajali*, ed. P.Y. Deshpande. Bern: Scherz.

Perlmutter, D. and Villoldo, A. (2011) *Power Up Your Brain*. London: Hay House.

Petzold, H. (1996) *Integrative Bewegungs- und Leibtherapie*. Paderborn: Junfermann.

Pitman, R.K., Altman, B., Greenwald, E., Longpre, R.E., Macklin, M.L., Poiré, R.E. *et al.* (1991) 'Psychiatric complications during flooding therapy for posttraumatic stress disorder.' *Journal of Clinial Psychiatry 52*, 1, 17–20.

Porges, S.W. (2011) *The Polyvagal Theory: Neuophysiological Foundation of Emotions, Attachment, Communication, and Self-Regulation*. London: W.W. Norton & Company.

Posner, M.I. and Rothbart, M.K. (2007) 'Research on attention networks as a model for the integration of psychological science.' *Annual Review of Psychology 58*, 1–23.

Putnam, F.W. (1997) *Dissociation in Children and Adolescents*. New York: Guilford Press.

Reddemann, L. (2001) *Imagination als heilsame Kraft. Zur Behandlung von Traumafolgen mit ressourcenorientierten Verfahren*. Stuttgart: Pfeiffer bei Klett-Cotta.

Resick, P.A. (2011) *Therapist's Manual—Cognitive Processing Therapy*. Veteran/Military Version. Available at www.psych.ryerson.ca/cptcanadastudy/CPT_Canada_Study/

Study_Materials_files/Basic%20Therapist%20Manual%20Text_title%20page%20
updated.pdf, accessed on 27 January 2017.

Resick, P.A. and Schnicke, M.K. (1993) *Cognitive Processing Therapy for Rape Victims.*
London: Sage Publications.

Rizzolatti, G. and Craighero, L.A. (2004) 'The mirror neuron system.' *Annual Review of
Neuroscience 27*, 169–92.

Rohnfeld, E. (2011) *Chair Yoga: Seated Exercises for Health and Wellbeing.* London: Singing
Dragon.

Rothschild, B. (2002) *The Body Remembers: The Psychophysiology of Trauma and Trauma
Treatment.* London: Norton Professional Books.

Rumi (1995) *The Essential Rumi.* Translated by Coleman Banks. London: Penguin.

Sachsse, U. and Roth, G. (2008) 'Die Integration neurobiologischer und psychoanalytischer
Ergebnisse in der Behandlung Traumatisierter.' In M. Leuzinger-Bohleber, G. Roth,
and A. Buchheim, *Psychoanalyse, Neurobiologie, Trauma.* Stuttgart: Schattauer.

Sageman, S. (2002) 'How SK Can Treat the Cognitive, Psychodynamic, and Neuropathic
Problems of Posttraumatic Stress Disorder.' Proceeding of the Science of Breath
International Symposium on 'Sudarshan Kriya, Pranayama and Consciousness'.
March. New Delhi, India: All India Institute of Medical Sciences.

Sageman, S. (2004) 'Breaking through the despair: Spiritually oriented group therapy as
a means of healing women with severe mental illness.' *Journal of the American Academy
of Psychoanalysis and Dynamic Psychiatry 32*, 125–41.

Salmon, P., Sephton, S., Weissbecker, I., Hoover, K., Ulmer, C., and Studts, J.L. (2004)
'Mindfulness meditation in clinical practice.' *Cognitive and Behavioral Practice 11*,
434–46.

Santorelli, S. (1999) *Heal Thy Self: Lessons on Mindfulness in Medicine.* New York: Random
House.

Saraswati, Swami Satyananda (2010) *Asana, Pranayama, Mudra and Bandha.* Cologne:
Ananda Verlag.

Sass, H., Wittchen, H.-U., and Zaudig, M. (2003) *Diagnostisches und Statistisches Manual
Psychischer Störungen.* Göttingen: Hogrefe.

Schauer, M. and Elbert, T. (2010) 'Dissociation following traumatic stress, etiology and
treatment.' *Zeitschrift für Psychologie 218*(2), 109–27.

Schauer, M., Neuner, F., and Elbert, T. (2011) *Narrative Exposure Therapy: A Short-Term
Treatment for Traumatic Stress Disorders.* Göttingen: Hogrefe.

Schore, A. (2008) 'Modern attachment theory: The central role of affect regulation in
development and treatment.' *Clinical Social Work Journal 36*, 9–20.

Schreiber-Willnow, K. and Hertel, G. (eds) (2006) *Rhein-Klinik: Aufsätze aus dem Innenleben.*
Frankfurt: VAS-Verlag, pp.157–71.

Segal, Z., Williams, J.M., and Teasdale, J. (2002) *Mindfulness-based Cognitive Therapy for
Depression.* New York: Guilford Press.

Shapiro, S.L., Carlson, L.E., Astin, J.A., and Freedman, B. (2006) 'Mechanisms of
mindfulness.' *Journal of Clinical Psychology 62*, 373–86.

Stankovic, L. (2011) 'Transforming trauma: A qualitative feasibility study of integrative
restoration (iRest) yoga nidra on combat-related post-traumatic stress disorder.'
International Journal of Yoga Therapy 21(1), 23–37.

Steele, B.F. (1994) 'Psychoanalysis and the maltreatment of children.' *Journal of the
American Psychoanalytic Association 42*, 1001–25.

Stern, D.N. (1985) *The Interpersonal World of the Infant.* New York: Basic Books.

Stolbach, B. (2007) 'Developmental trauma disorder: A new diagnosis for children affected by complex trauma.' *International Society for the Study of Trauma and Dissociation News 25*(6), 4–6.

Streeter, C.C., Jensen, E.J., Permutter, R.M., Cabral, H.J. *et al.* (2007) 'Yoga Asana sessions increase brain GABA levels: A pilot study.' *Journal of Alternative and Complementary Medicine 13*(4), 419–26.

Streeter, C.C., Whitfield, Th.H., Owen, L., Rein, T. *et al.* (2010) 'Effects of yoga versus walking on mood, anxiety, and brain GABA levels: A randomized controlled MRS study.' *Journal of Alternative and Complementary Medicine 16*(11), 1145–52.

Telles, S. and Desiraju, T. (1991) 'Oxygen consumption during pranayamic type of very slow-rate breathing.' *Indian Journal of Medical Research 94*, 357–63.

Telles, S. and Desiraju, T. (1992) 'Heart rate alterations in different types of pranayama.' *Indian Journal of Physiology and Pharmacology 36*, 287–88.

Telles, S. and Naveen, K.V. (2008) 'Voluntary breath regulation in yoga: Its relevance and physiological effects.' *Biofeedback 36*(2), 70–3.

Telles, S., Naveen, K.V., and Dash M. (2007) *Yoga Reduces Symptoms of Distress in Tsunami Survivors in the Andaman Islands.* Bangalore, India: Swami Vivekananda Yoga Research Foundation (A Yoga University).

Telles, S., Singh, N., and Balkrishna, A. (2011) 'Managing mental health disorders resulting from trauma through yoga: A review.' *Depression Research and Treatment 2012*, Article ID 401513.

Telles, S., Joshi, M., Dash, M., Raghuraj, P., Naveen, K.V., and Nagendra, H.R. (2004) 'An evaluation of the ability to voluntarily reduce the heart rate after a month of yoga practice.' *Integrative Physiological & Behavioral Science 39*(2), 119–25.

US Department of Veterans Affairs (no date) 'PTSD and DSM-5.' Available at www.ptsd.va.gov/professional/PTSD-overview/dsm5_criteria_ptsd.asp, accessed on 6 January 2017.

Vaiva, G., Thomas, P., Ducrocq, F., Fontaine, M. *et al.* (2004) 'Low post-trauma GABA plasma levels as a predictive factor in the development of acute post-traumatic stress disorder.' *Biological Psychiatry 55*, 250–54.

van der Kolk, B.A. (2005) 'Developmental Trauma Disorder.' *Psychiatric Annals*, pp.401–8.

van der Kolk, B.A. (2009) 'Yoga and Post-Traumatic Stress Disorder: Interview, M.D.' *Integral Yoga Magazine*, pp.12–13.

van der Kolk, B.A. and Jehuda, R. (2009) 'Trauma-sensitive yoga: Principles, practice, and research.' *International Journal of Yoga Therapy 19*(1), 123–28.

van der Kolk, B.A., Burbridge, J.A., and Suzuki, J. (1997) 'The psychobiology of traumatic memory: Clinical implications of neuroimaging studies.' *Annals of the New York Academy of Science 821*, 99–113.

van der Kolk, B.A., Fisler, R.E., and Bloom, S.L. (1996) 'Dissociation and fragmentary nature of traumatic memories.' *British Journal of Psychotherapy 12*, 352–66.

van der Kolk, B.A., McFarlane, A., and Weisaeth, L. (2006) *Traumatic Stress: The Effects of Overwhelming Experience on Mind, Body, and Society.* New York: The Guilford Press.

van der Kolk, B.A., Stone, L., West, J., Rhodes, A. *et al.* (2014) 'Yoga as an adjunctive treatment for posttraumatic stress disorder: A randomized controlled trial.' *Journal of Clinical Psychiatry 75*(6), 59–65.

Waelde, L.C., Thompson, L., and Gallagher-Thompson, D. (2004) 'A pilot study of yoga and meditation intervention for dementia caregiver stress.' *Journal of Clinical Psychology 60*(6), 677–87.

Walsh, R. and Shapiro, S L. (2006) 'The meeting of meditative disciplines and western psychology: A mutually enriching dialogue.' *American Psychologist 61*, 227–39.

Wessa, M. and Flor, H. (2002) 'Posttraumatische Belastungsstörungen und Traumagedächtnis—Eine psychobiologische Perspektive.' *Zeitschrift für Psychosomatische Medizin und Psychotherapie 48*, 28–37.

West, J. (2011) 'Moving to Heal: Women's Experiences of Therapeutic Yoga after Complex Trauma.' Dissertation. Available at https://static1.squarespace.com/static/56053860e4b068a8e5d5caf8/t/56d040ab1d07c08478c6532f/1456488628289/Moving+to+Heal.pdf, accessed on 27 January 2017.

Wöller, W. (2006) *Trauma und Persönlichkeitsstörungen.* Stuttgart: Schattauer.

Zeidler, W. (2007) 'Unterschiede in der Emotionsverarbeitung bei Achtsamkeitsmeditierenden und Nichtmeditierenden—Eine Startle-Studie.' Unpublished diploma thesis. Institute for Psychology and Ergonomics at the Technical University of Berlin.

SUBJECT INDEX

choices, emphasis on 149–52
    example for offering choice 151–2
cingulate cortex, brain 20
cognitive processing
    limitations of 49–50
    top down versus bottom up approach 56
Cognitive Processing Therapy (CPT) 58
cognitive therapy 48
cognitive-verbal interventions, and yoga 96–7
coherent breathing 210–11
combat fatigue 31
complex PTSD 22, 33–4, 36, 37–9, 47, 115
    therapeutic relationship 69
concentration 81, 88–9, 240
consciousness, contents of 218–19
contact, making (handout) 285
contemplation 82
contentment 79, 80
conversational therapy 97
corrections 152–4
cortex, brain 45, 46
    frontal lobes 61
cortisol 35

dance therapy 93
decision-making, freedom in 149–52
defensive actions, unfinished 64
delta fibers, neural pathways 251
depression 57, 106
developmental traumas 29, 30, 36, 41
dharana (concentration) 81, 88–9, 240
dhyana (meditation) 81, 82
*Diagnostic and Statistical Manual of Mental
    Disorders*, 5th edition (DSM-5) 27–8
    PTSD included in 31
Dialectic-Behavioral Therapy (DBT) 98
diaphragm 199–200
    diaphragmatic breathing, relaxed 201, 203
diencephalon 45
differentiation
    learning to differentiate 245–7
    trauma therapy 116
disgust 28, 41, 65, 234
disorders, causes 57–8
dissociation 17, 40–2, 53
    fight, flight or freeze reaction 51
    and flashback 268–70
    negative attributes 42
    positive symptoms 42
    somatoform dissociation 32, 41–2
dorsal vagal reactions 54
Downward Dog Pose 196–8, 269, 270
dreams, recurring 32
dual representation theory 46

ego strengthening 58
Eightfold Path, of Raja yoga 77–82, 88, 89
embodiment 19
    see also body
Emerson, D.
    Overcoming Trauma Through Yoga 268
    Trauma-Sensitive Yoga 98
    see also author index
emotions
    processing of 56, 100
    regulation of 107–8
    role 60–1
empowerment, sense of 21, 22
    empowerment language 154–5
    self-empowerment 41
energy discharge 51
enlightenment 81, 86
enteroception, becoming familiar with 162
equals, relationship of 264–8
executive attention 107
exhalation, prolonged 104, 206
    with Alternative Breath 215
    and mindfulness 222
    with Sun Breath 212
exposure therapy 66–7
    body-oriented approach 22
    and/or yoga 95–6
exteroception 61

fainting 28, 40, 41, 44
    fear of 207
fast breathing 104, 119, 209
fear response
    breathing in an emotional stupor 204–5
    constant feelings of fear 206
    inappropriately fearful behavior 64
    information processing, hierarchy 46, 47
    network 233, 260
fight-or-flight reaction 20, 43–4, 50–3, 205
five *niyamas* 79–80, 83
five *yamas* 78–9, 83
flaccid immobility 41, 44, 195
flashbacks 17, 32, 268–70
    physical 40
forward bends 133, 162, 170–1, 191–2
freezing 51, 55, 235
    see also fight, flight or freeze reaction

gamma-aminobutyric acid (GABA) 94
gender factors, experiences of trauma 28
"general nervous shock" 31
glutamate transmission 94
goals and values, clarification 219
God, trust in 79

Author Index

CPI Antony Rowe

Chippenham, UK

2019-03-13 12:12